# I Messed Around and Figured Out

# My Worth

by
Sarah Ruth Latham

ISBN: 9781960853226

Painting Credit: Brittany Deanes of Brittany World
Studios

Liberation's Publishing House – Columbus. MS

# I Messed Around and Figured Out

## My Worth

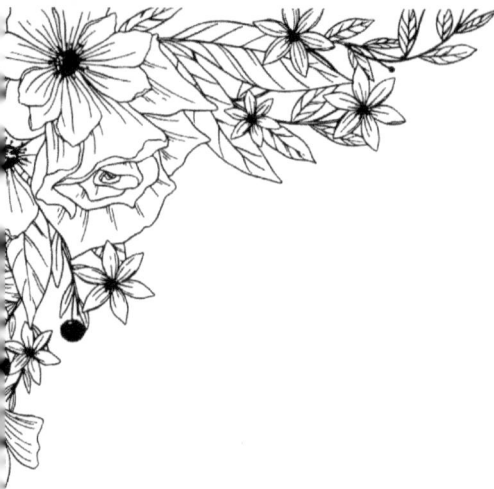

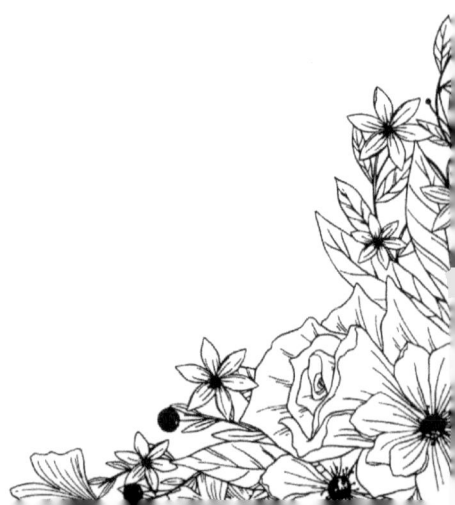

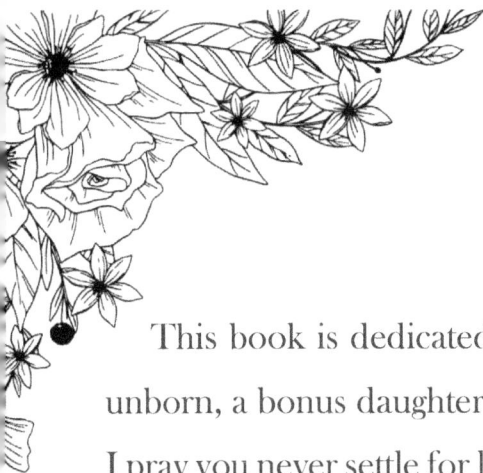

This book is dedicated to my daughter, whether unborn, a bonus daughter, or waiting to be adopted, I pray you never settle for less. Always know that your worth is based on how you see yourself. Love yourself. Honor yourself. Protect yourself. Mama promises to be there to help you figure it out! I love you.

A special dedication to J + A, my clients, who lovingly "cyber stalked" me and encouraged me to turn my self-love posts, from Instagram and Facebook, into a book!

Lastly, thank you to Q. You showed me that I needed to refocus on myself because I had lost my way. "You are every inspiration and every joy to me. Siempre Nosotras."

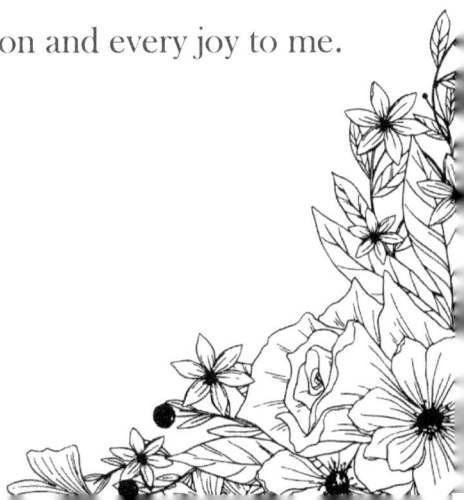

# Introduction

This book encompasses four main components:

1. Things I wish I had known before my self-love journey.

2. Things I have learned and felt while traveling on my own journey, so far! I am still learning and still traveling.

3. Reminders for those on their self-love journeys, no matter what stage of the journey is being traveled through.

4. Encouragement to never mess around and forget your worth.

This book is everyday inspiration, motivation, and encouragement for the self-loving travelers who are on their self-love journeys.

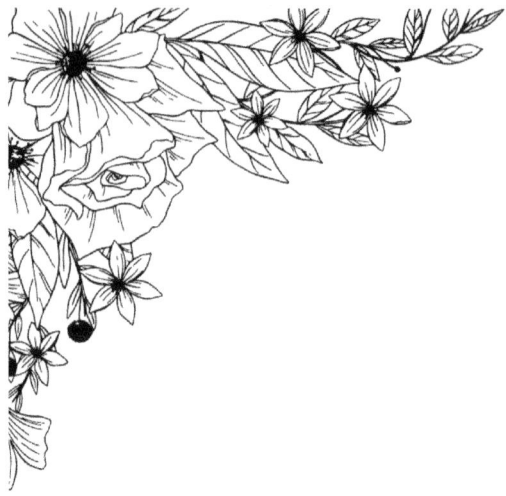

Welcome Back My Self-Loving Travelers...

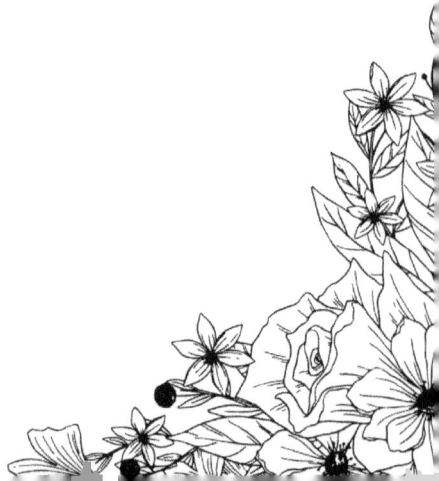

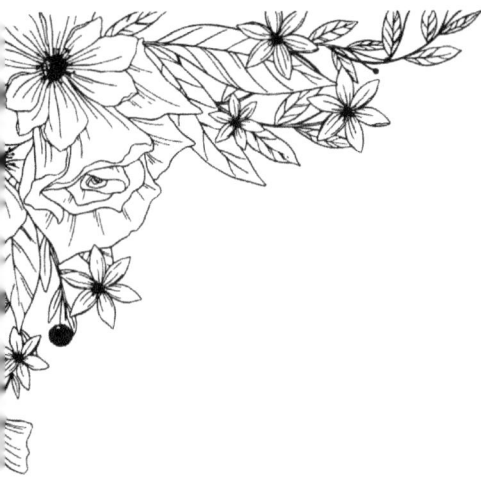

You will never be enough for someone else until you are enough for yourself

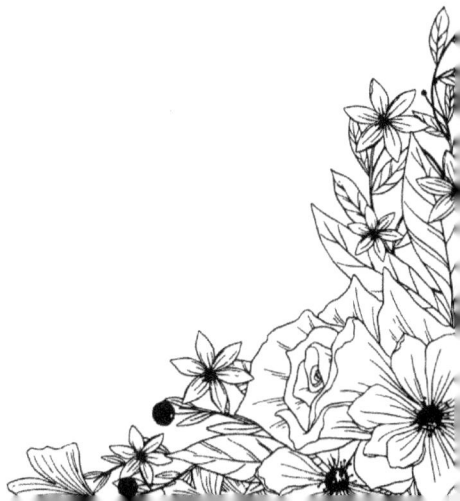

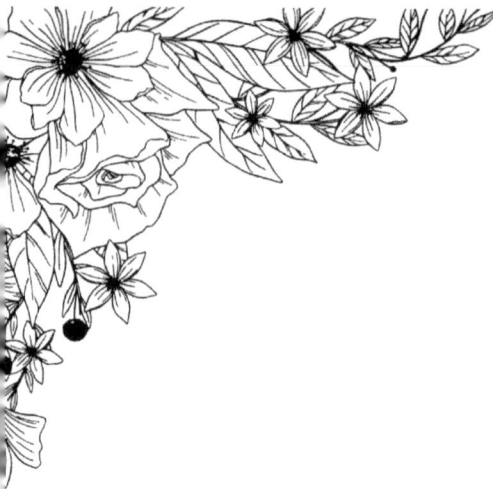

I was tired of heartbreak, so I decided to give my heart a break.

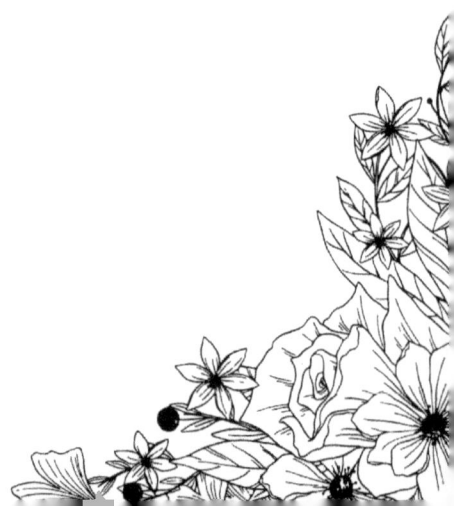

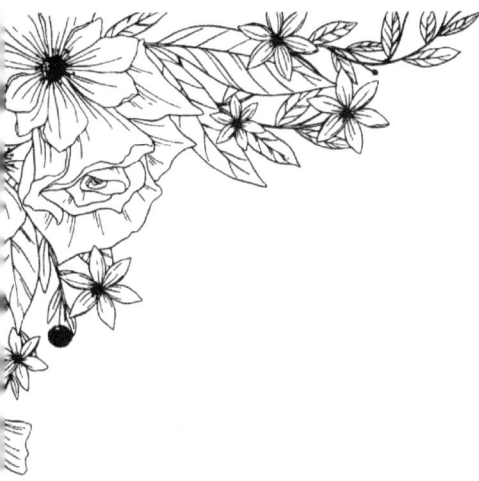

You cannot be the light to someone who chooses to live in darkness.

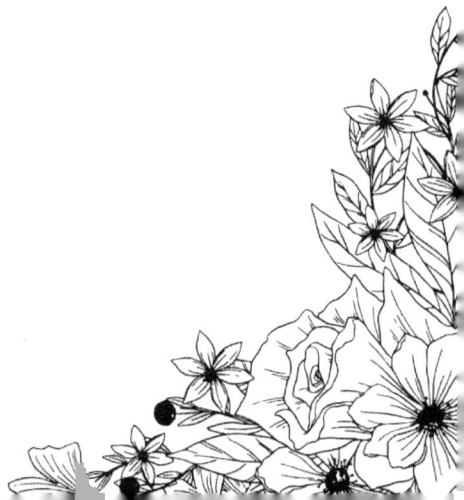

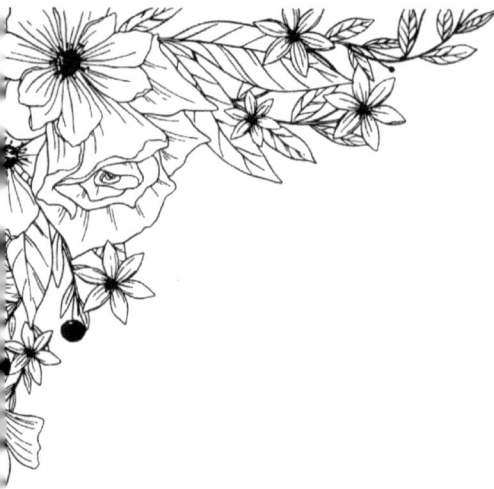

**Food For Thought:** For as long as I can remember, I have always wanted someone in my life to experience my journey with me. However, it never worked out. I have realized that where I am in my journey, there is no room for anyone, but God and myself.

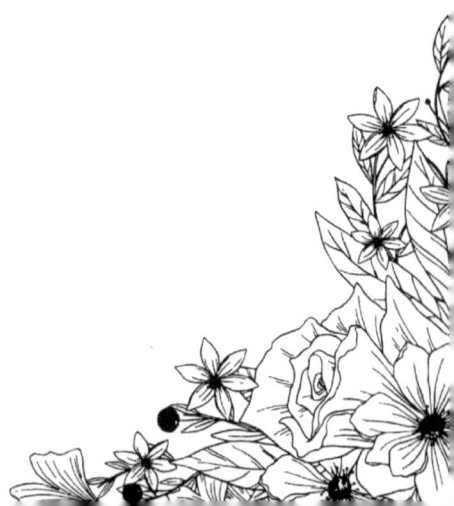

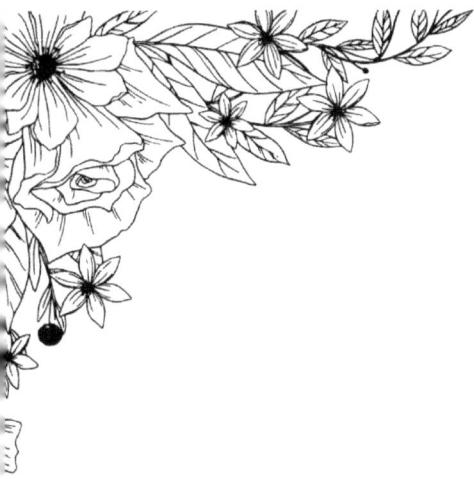

God has me on a path that is only for me. As I walk where He directs my steps, I know He is leading me to my purpose in life and to a love story that only God himself can write.

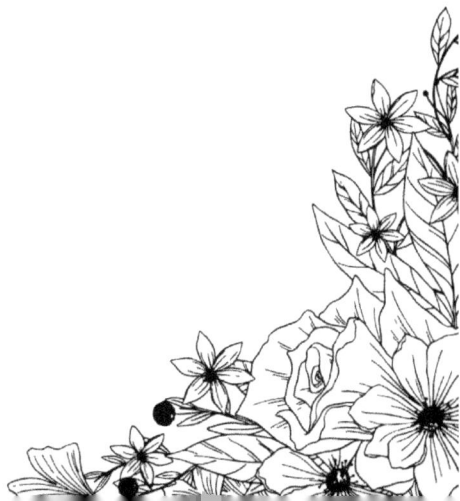

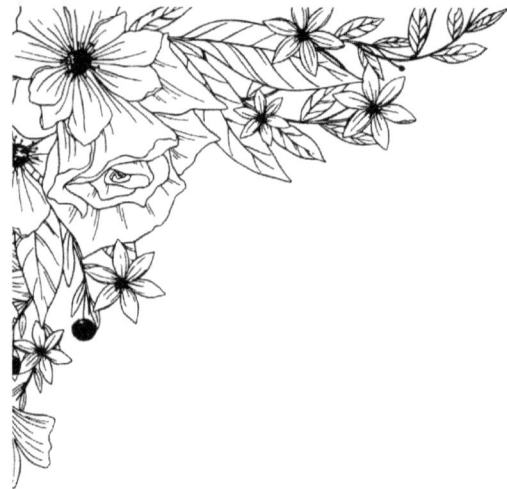

You cannot survive off of emotional breadcrumbs.
Darling, you need soul food.

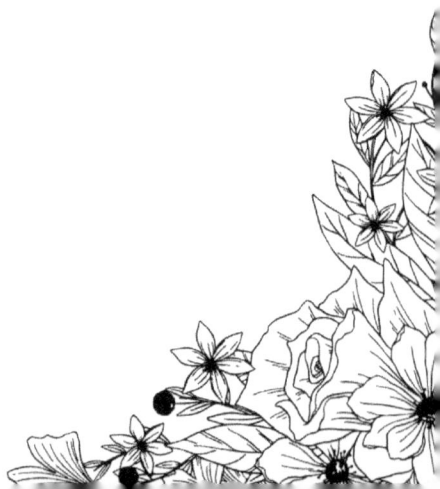

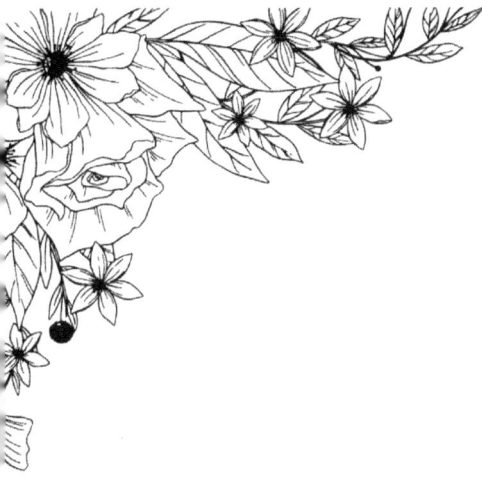

Love will ALWAYS live here.
With or without anyone else.

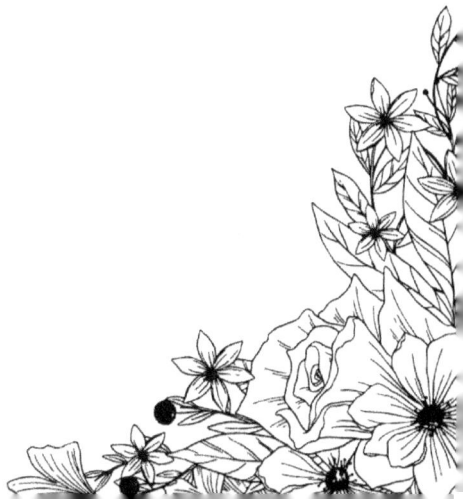

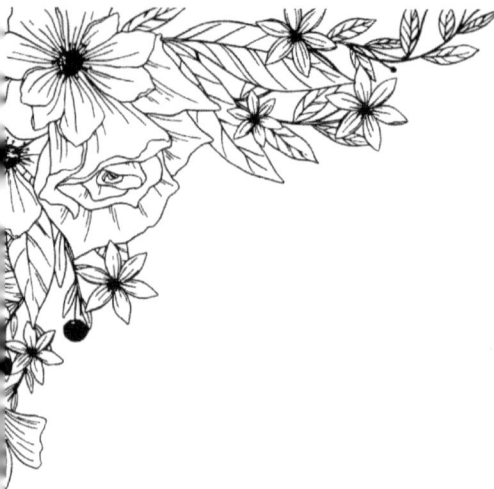

It is solely your responsibility to make sure you
receive the love you deserve.

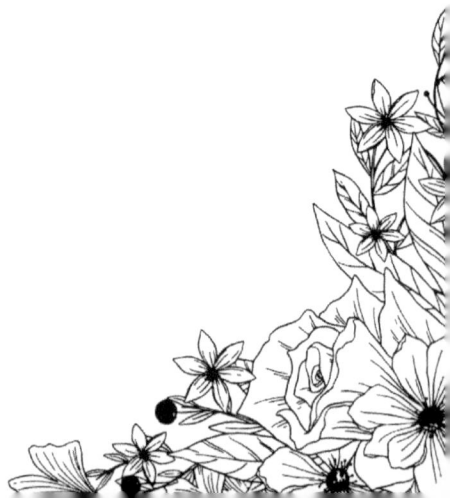

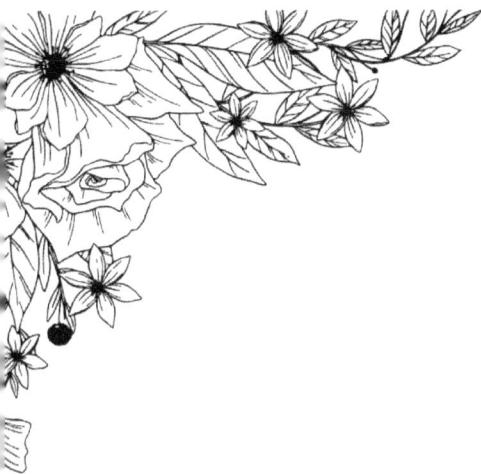

You cannot find someone, if you, yourself, are lost!

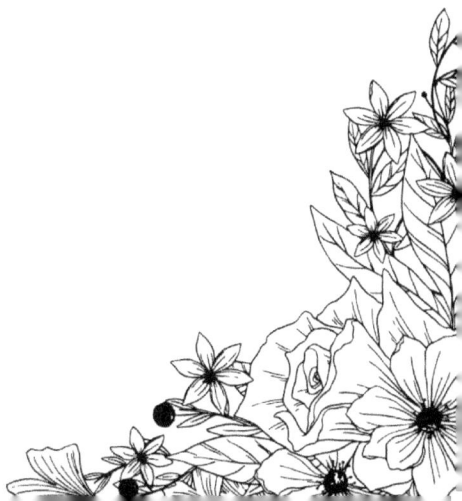

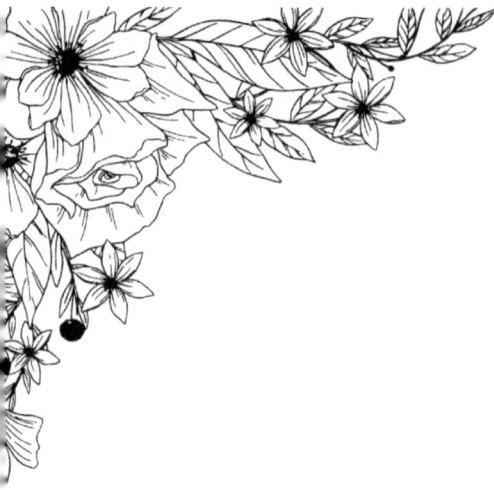

It is impossible to spell evolve without the letters found in LOVE, so while you evolve make sure to show yourself some love!

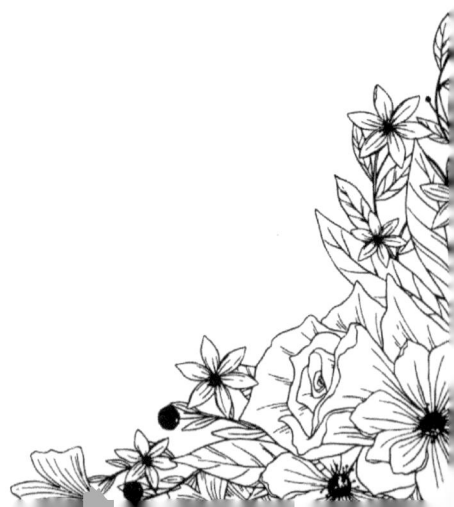

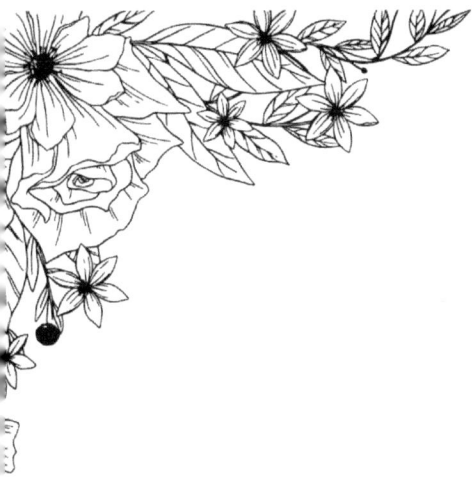

You must first heal before moving on. If you do not heal, then all you will have to offer is recycled hurt.

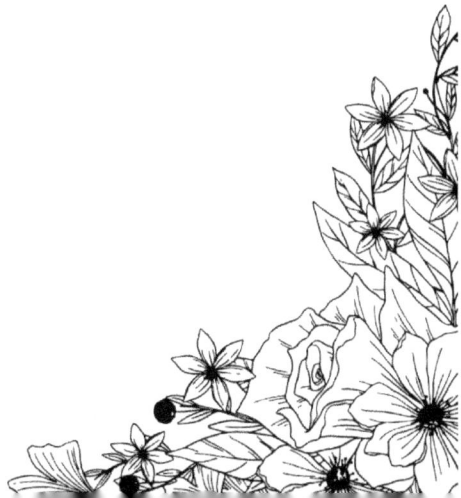

## The first year on my self-love journey

Months 1-3: I really wrestled with what I had done wrong, and if I could have done anything differently to fix the situation. This was a difficult transition for me. Here I was coming out of a place where I had always been told I was wrong or made to feel like I was not enough, so I was still in that mindset.

Months 4-6: I realized that I did all I could, and it was time for me to love myself the way I deserved. I immersed myself in God and His love for me. I began to realize that singleness was not a curse but a blessing. I started dating myself and figuring out who I was. I realized that I am funny when I want to be. I love how I look when my hair is huge. I adore colorful clothes. Random things I never knew because I was too focused on someone else.

Months 7-9: I started going out more alone and with friends. Began spending quality time with people I had neglected due to the toxic relationship I was in. I began laughing more and understanding what happiness and self-love truly meant.

Months 10-12: I was completely amazed at how good God was. I was happy that He held me through this tough process. I came out happier and more content. I realized that I could be alone and be okay.

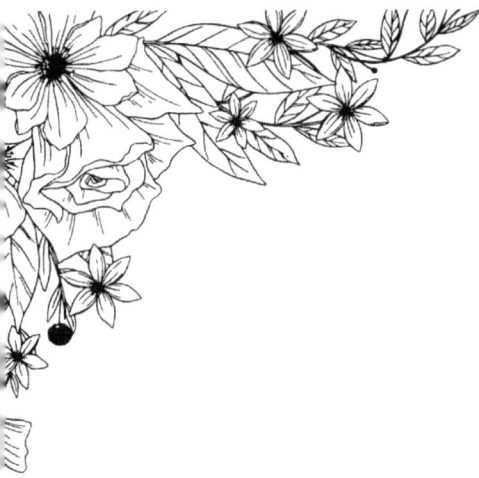

She wanted to know what a touch full of love felt like.

She wanted to know what a kiss full of love felt like.

She wanted to know what a relationship full of love felt like.

She wanted to know what love felt like.

So, she gave herself permission to love herself.

And she now knows she can experience the other things because she now understands love and experiences it every day.

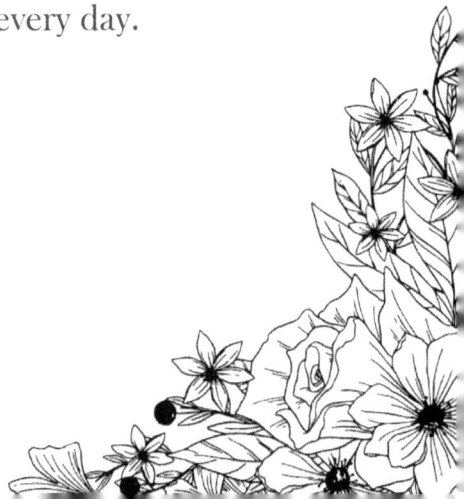

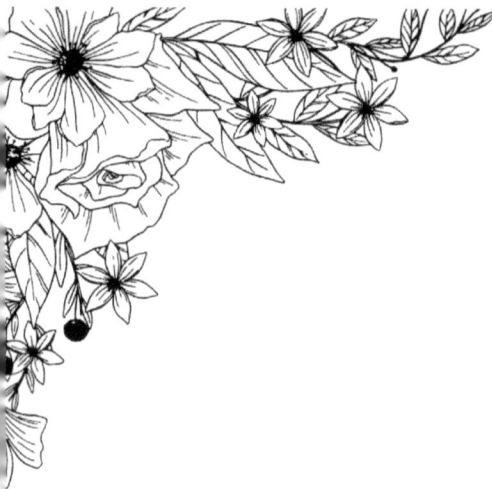

I read a quote in the early stages of my journey that stated, "being in love is like two dreamers dreaming the exact same dream". I hope that when love visits you again, it is coming from someone who is dreaming the exact same dream as you!

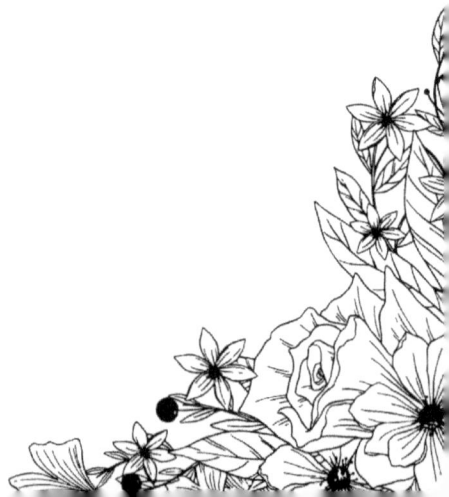

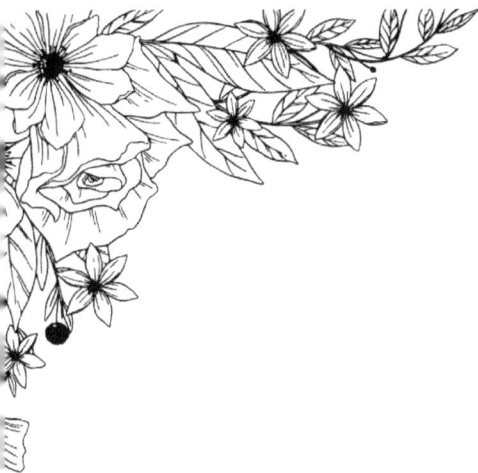

To whom it may concern,

If you see a person who is educated, independent, living their best life, striving for greatness, staying in their own lane, loving themselves, caring for themselves, and basically killing every aspect of the game. I have one piece of advice for you. If you have nothing of value or substance to add to them, then LEAVE THEM ALONE.

Thank you greatly for your

cooperation.

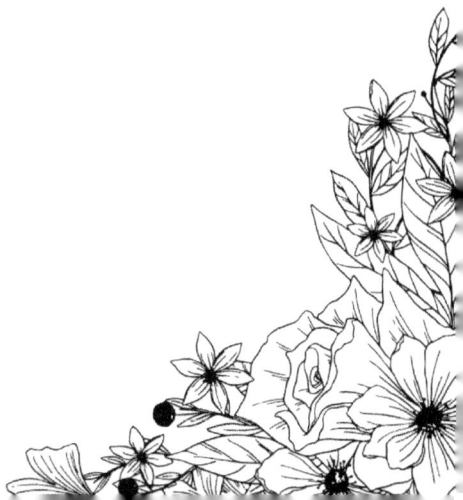

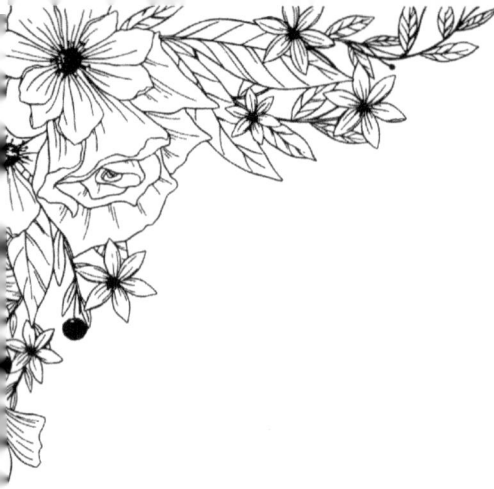

One day you will wake up, and the memories of that certain person will no longer matter or exist. That is when you will know that you have been healing. Until that time, do not beat yourself up through the process. People come, people go, but you will always have yourself. Take some time to invest in your healing. Everyone and everything will just have to wait!

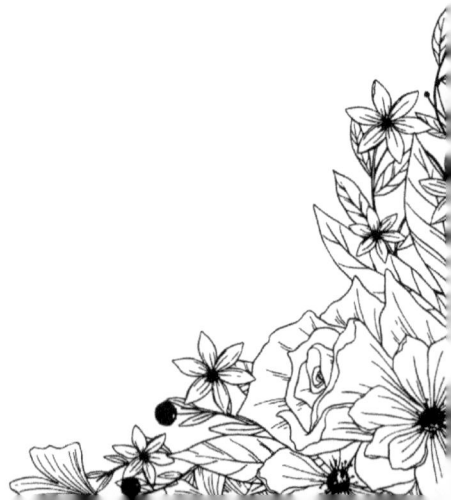

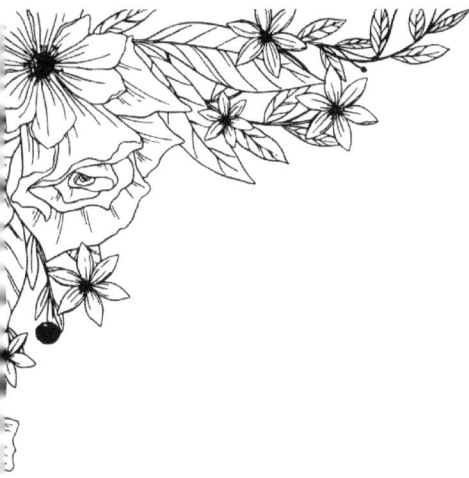

Chase your dreams, not a person! Your dreams will never betray you.

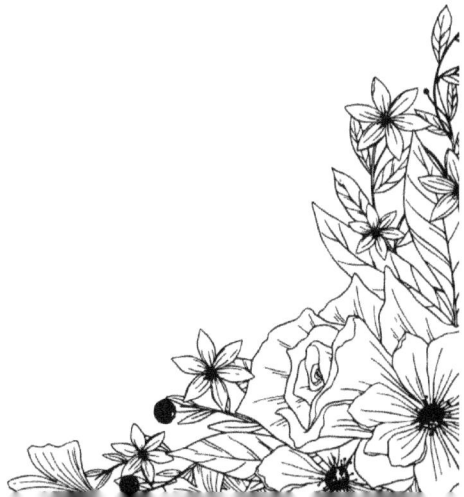

One cannot experience a **HEALthy** life, if they do not HEAL themselves first.

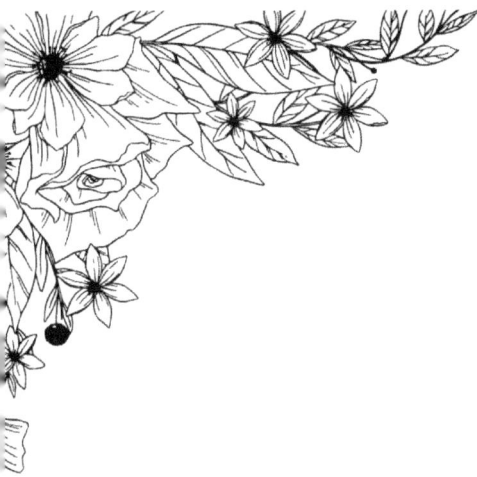

I am currently experiencing my season of healing! I do not know how long this season will last, and I do not care because it is very necessary. I am beyond excited to be here.

-replacing negative thoughts with positive thoughts is key to a successful self-love journey.

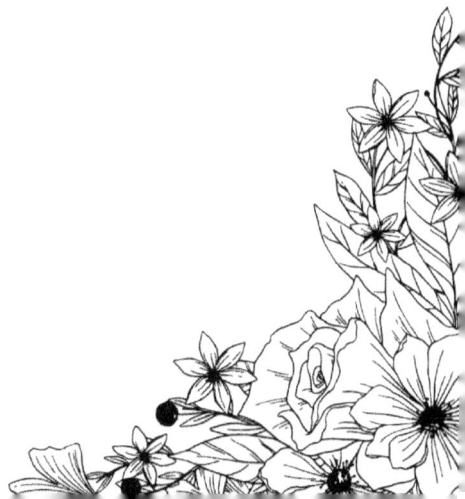

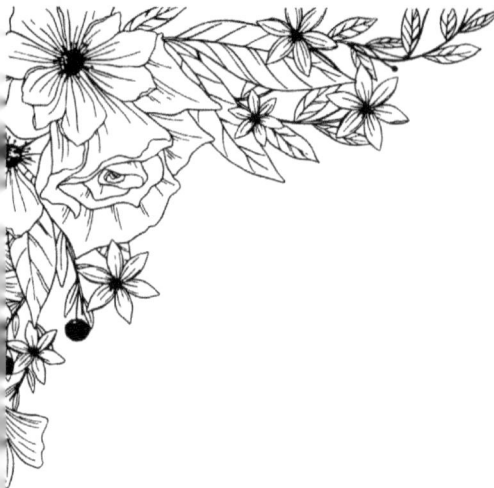

Most people stay in bad situations because it is familiar.

They are often afraid to take a chance on something foreign to them.

Trust me when I say... take that chance!

You will regret staying much more than you will regret leaving.

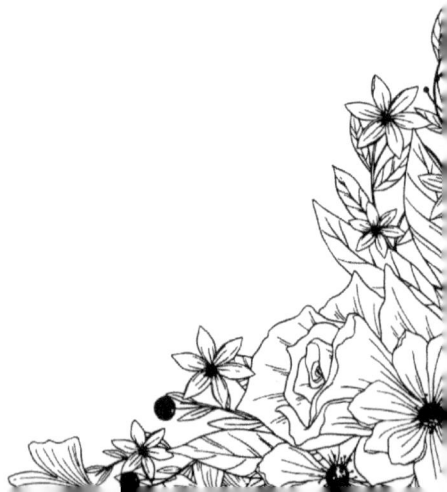

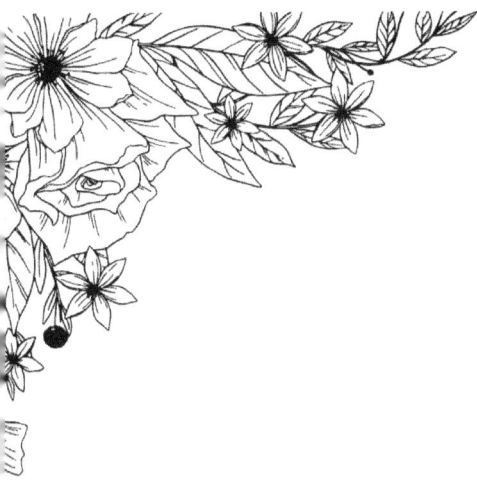

I would rather be alone for the rest of my life than spend my existence proving my worth to someone who is not even worthy of the worst parts of me!

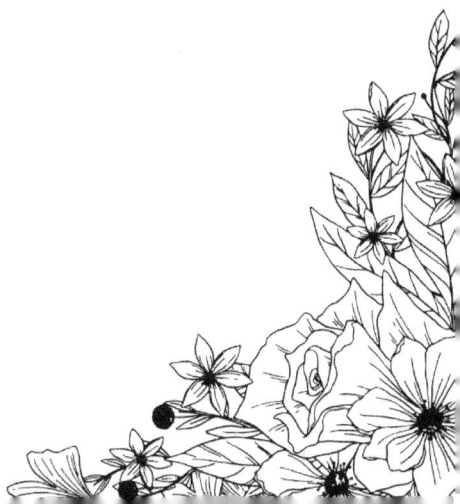

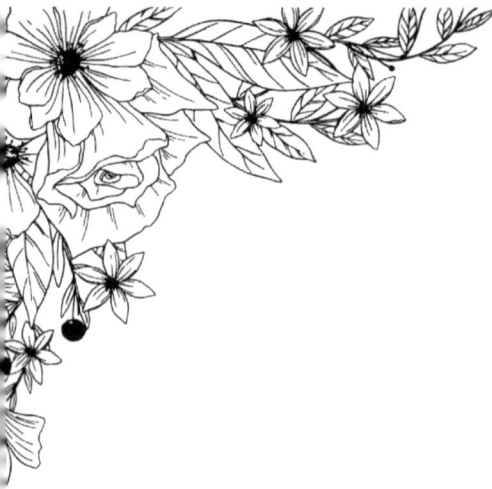

My hope, for the person reading this, is that you get EVERYTHING your heart desires.

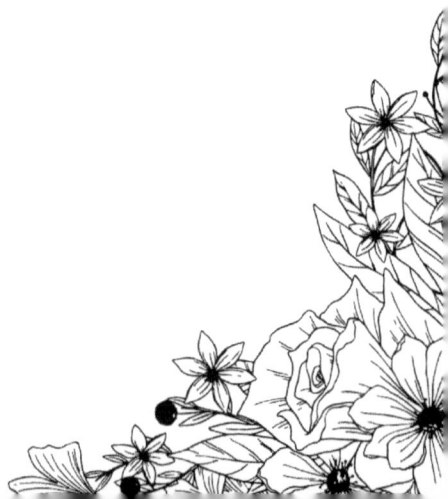

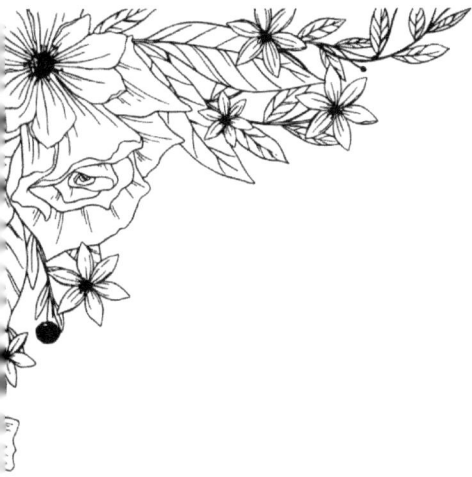

A lot of us need to understand that it is better to be alone and thriving than to be with someone who makes us feel like we are alone and dying.

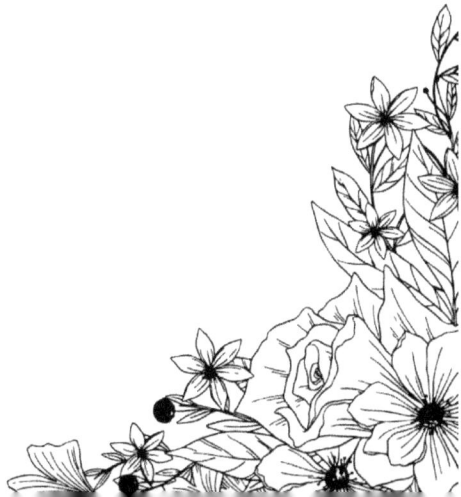

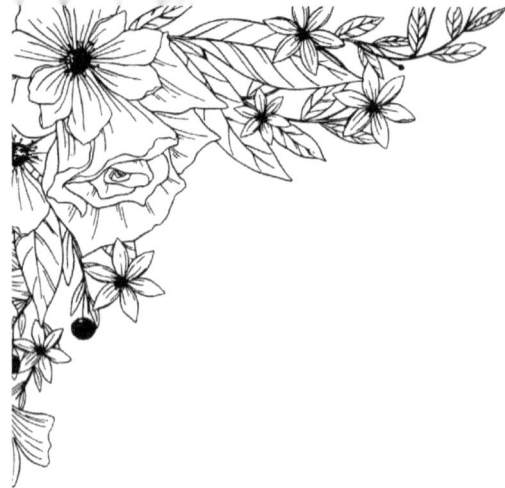

Do not allow your WANT for love to outweigh your NEED for respect.

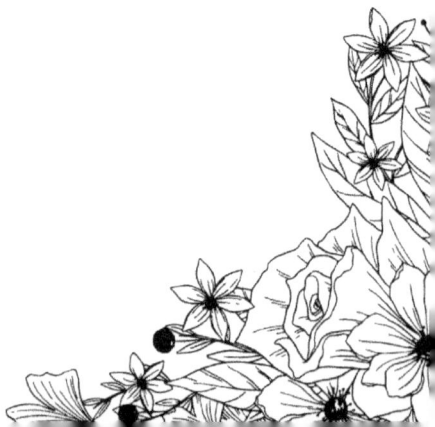

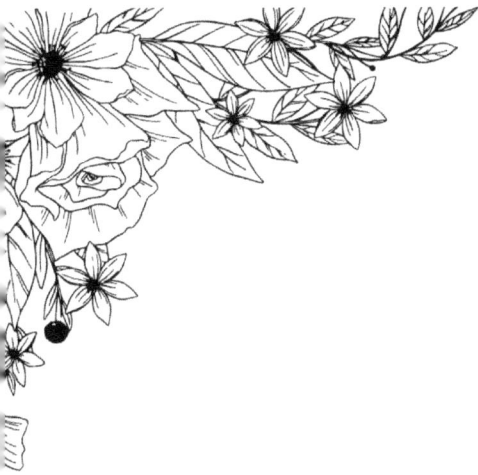

The loss of you was worth it because I ended up
finding myself in the process.

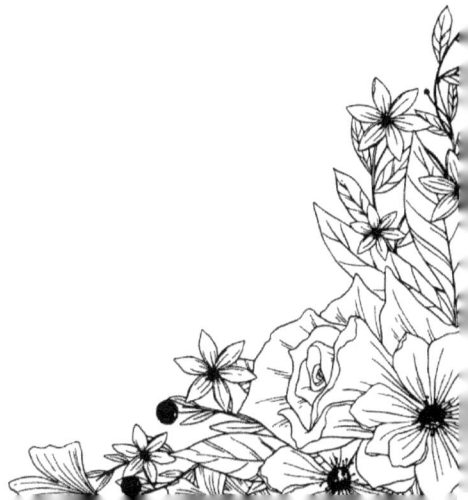

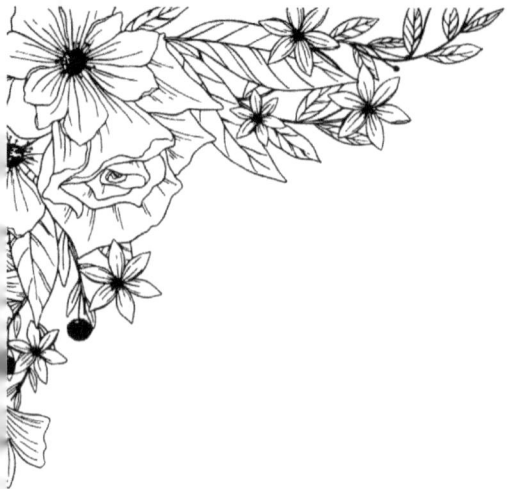

It is better to be picky than to be picked over!

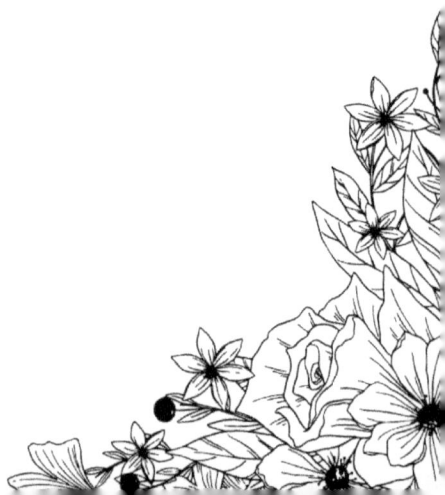

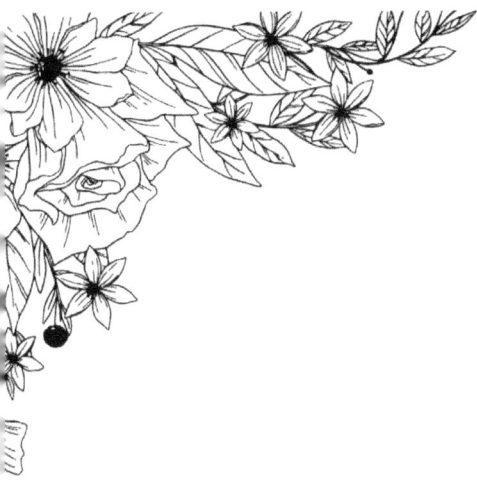

At no point in time should a person be allowed to claim you in private, while disowning you in public!

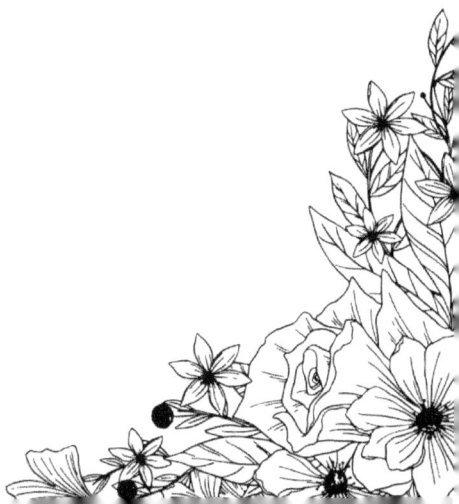

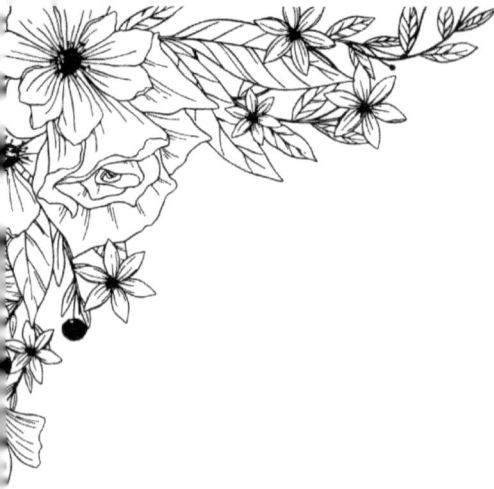

Even though you did not ask for forgiveness, I forgive you. May God bless your soul. Sincerely.

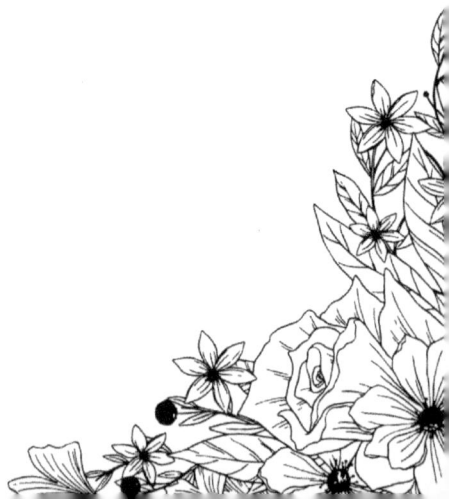

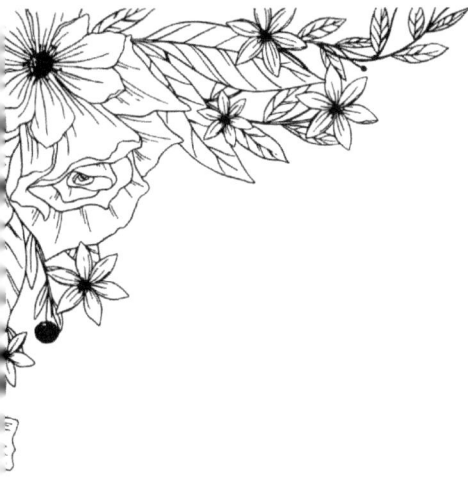

The love you accept from others is an indicator of
the love you show yourself.

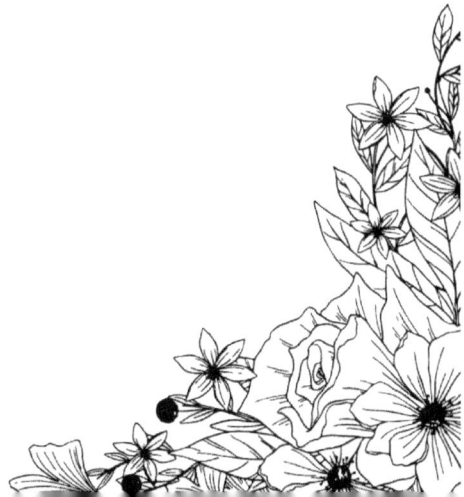

Whatever you choose to place your focus on is what will grow. I encourage you to CHOOSE WISELY.

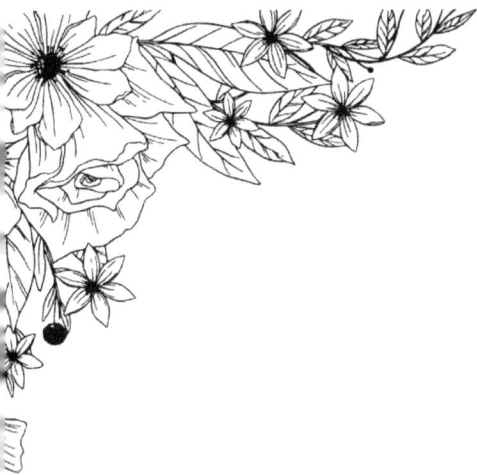

When you are too scared to let a person go, that is when you run the risk of being used and unhappy. If someone is not caring for you the way you deserve, you must let them go.

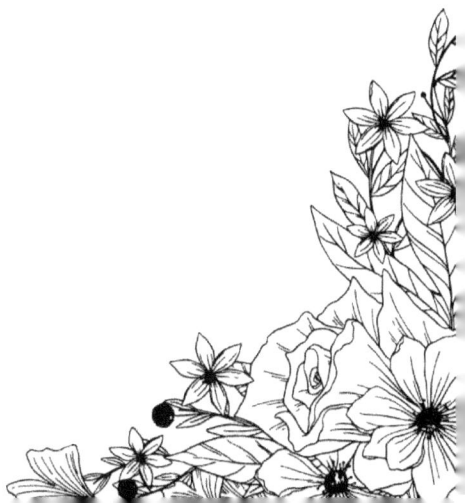

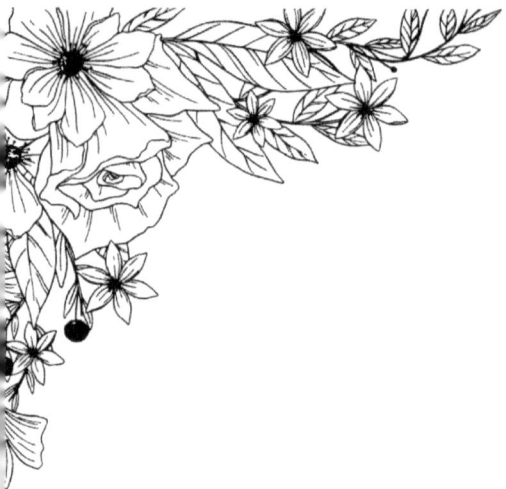

You must choose yourself above everything else.

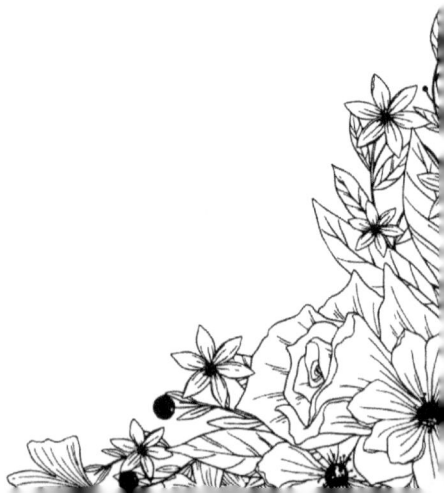

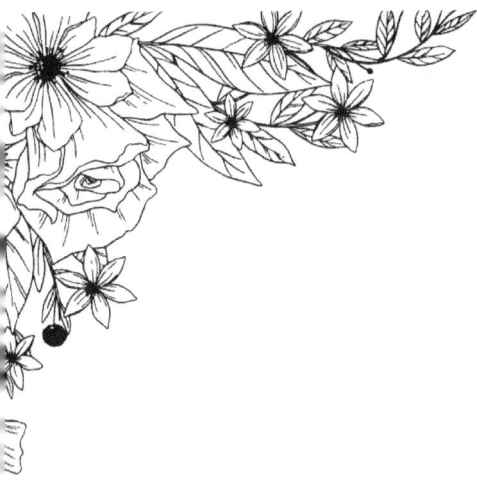

In this life we must sacrifice something we have always wanted for the belief that better is coming!

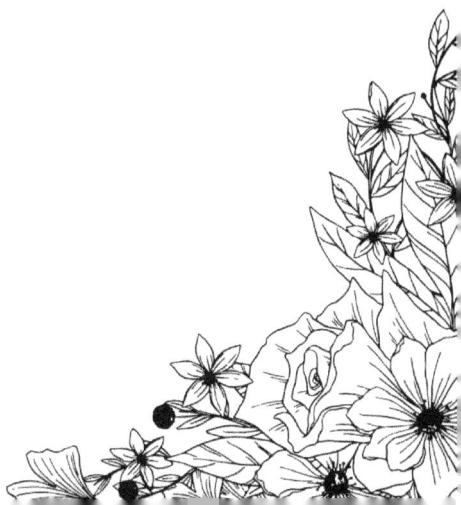

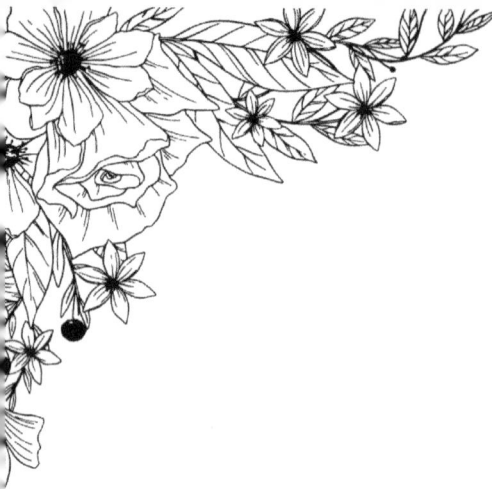

Stop giving your love away at a discounted rate.

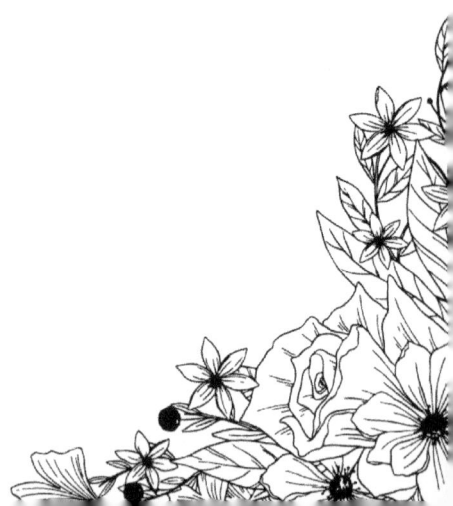

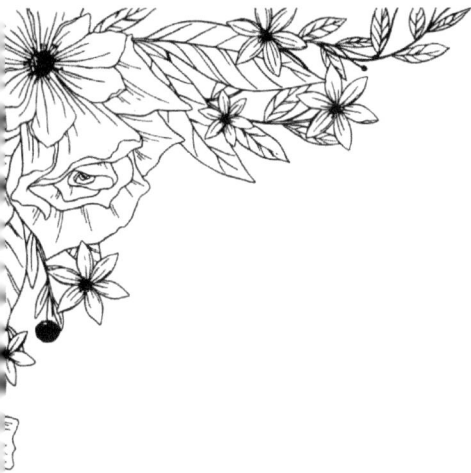

You are THE prize! Stop handing out quarters to everyone and giving them a chance to win you and your love.

The person who is meant to have you will bring their own quarters.

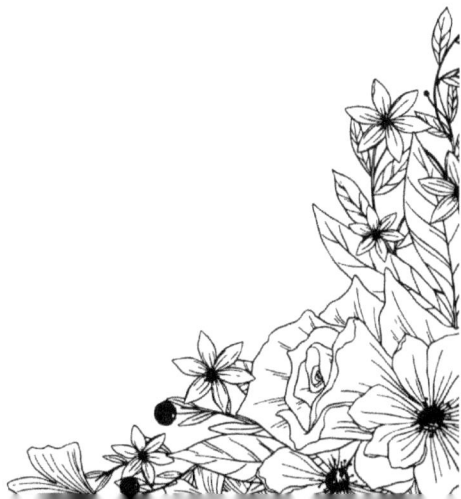

Who keeps telling people that the foundation of a relationship should be pain and toxicity?

Whoever it is, please stop it!

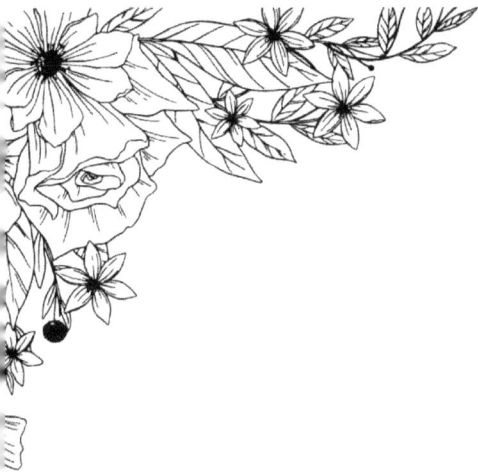

NO ONE is worth losing yourself over. You only get one you, so do not let anyone disturb your happiness and peace of mind.

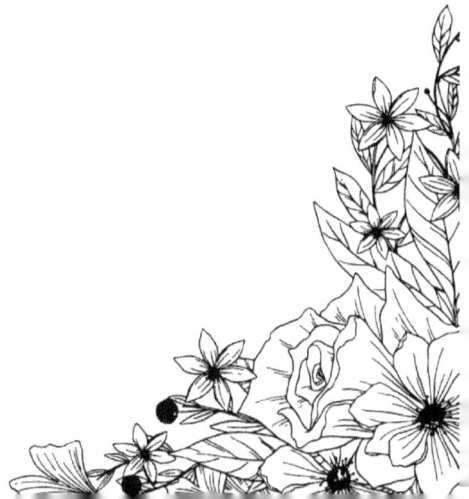

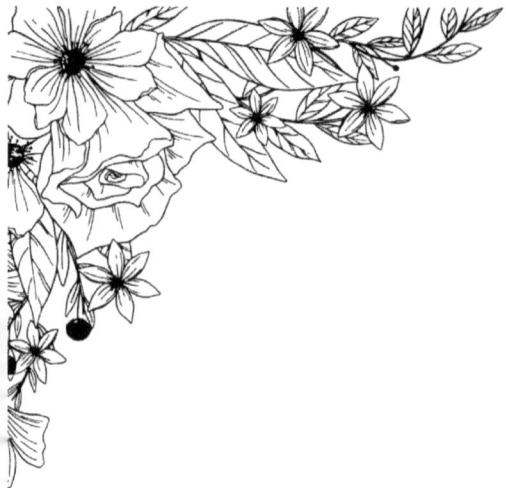

You cannot be seen as the magnificent person you are until you see yourself as the magnificent person you are.

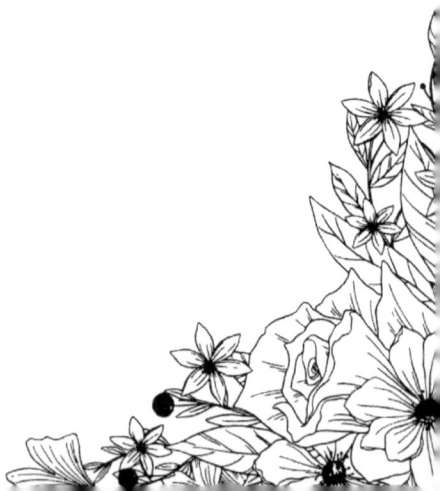

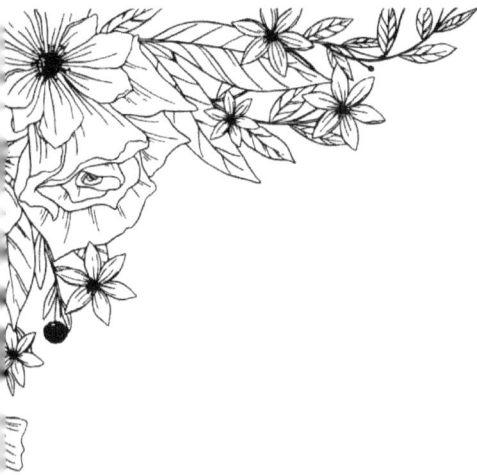

An emotionally unstable person will never know how to support you emotionally.

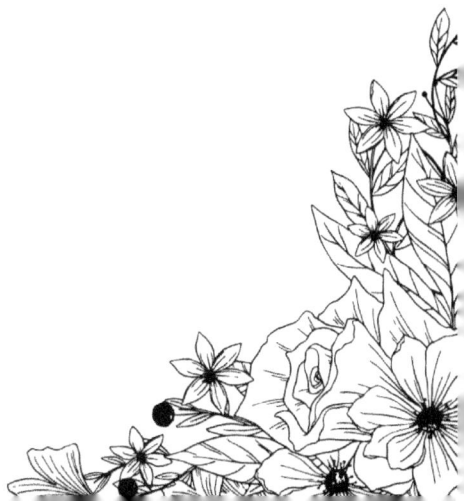

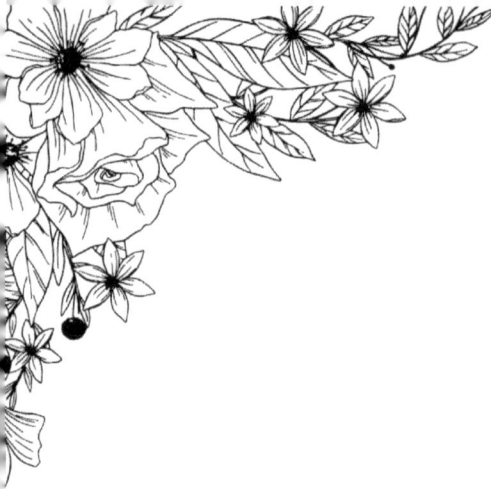

You cannot possibly know my story; it is not even
close to being finished.

Honestly, it is just getting started.

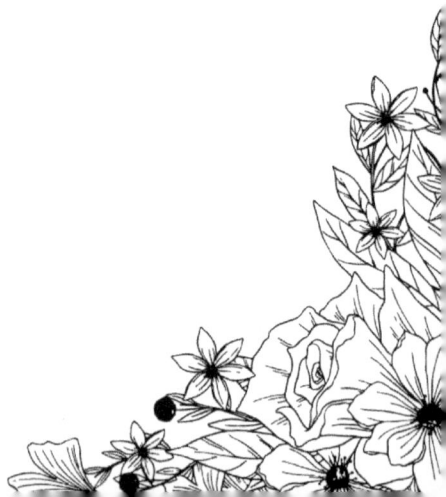

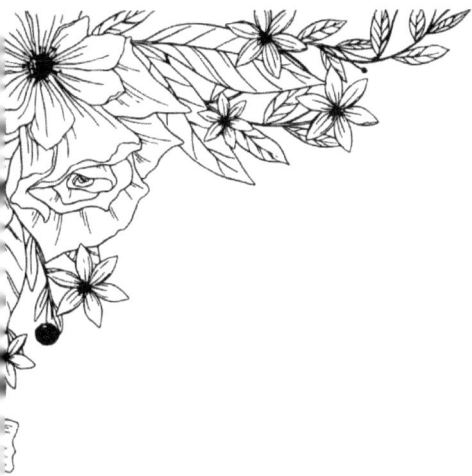

When drama continues to be the main course, it is time to move to a different table.

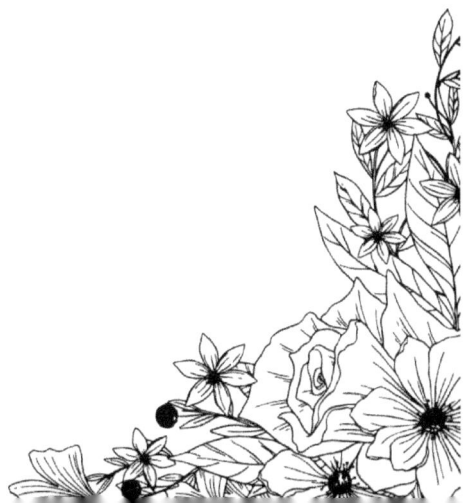

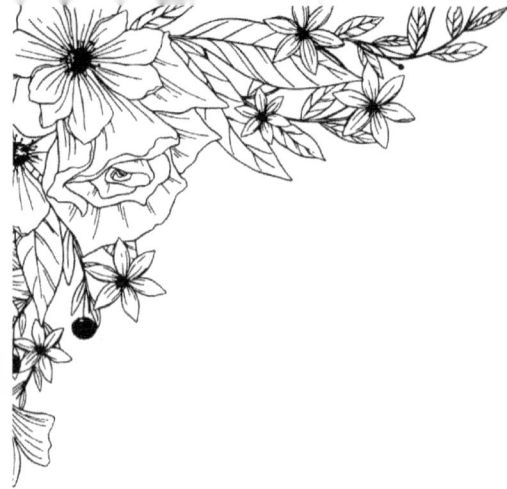

Do not allow someone to keep you a secret. We are too amazing to be kept secret.

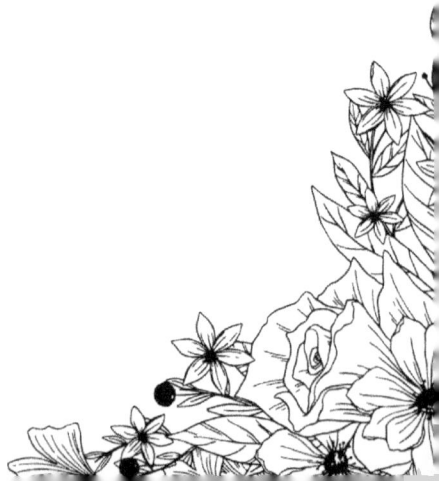

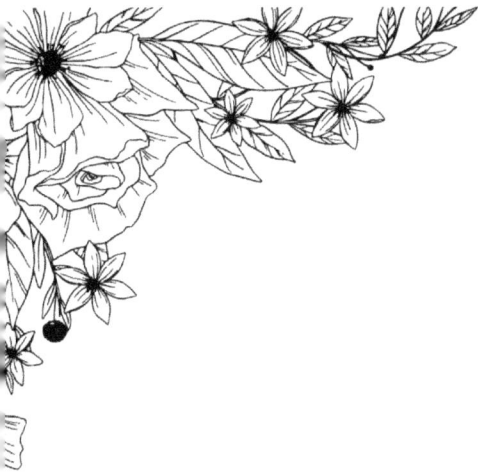

Why does it seem like having dysfunction in our relationships and lives is the only way to function?

We must learn to live peacefully and happily.

It is possible.

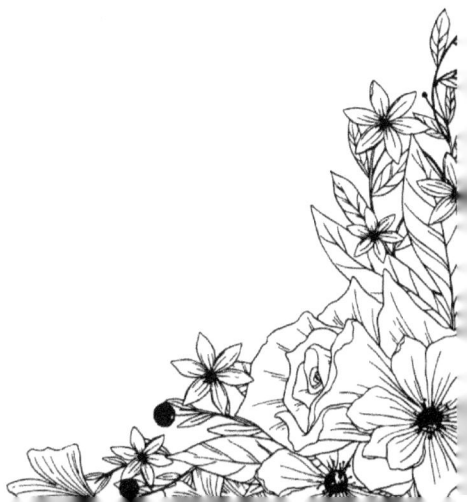

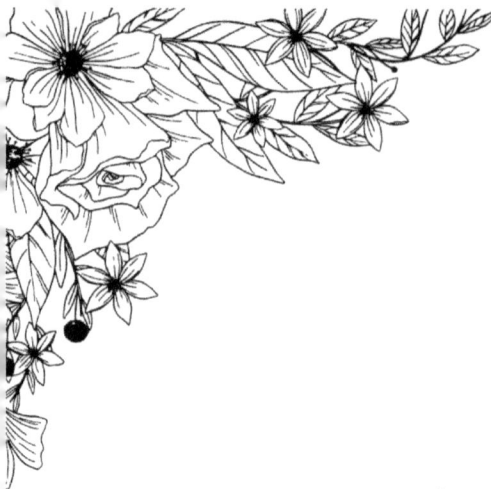

Now when I look in the mirror, I know what it means to have someone look at me with love in their eyes.

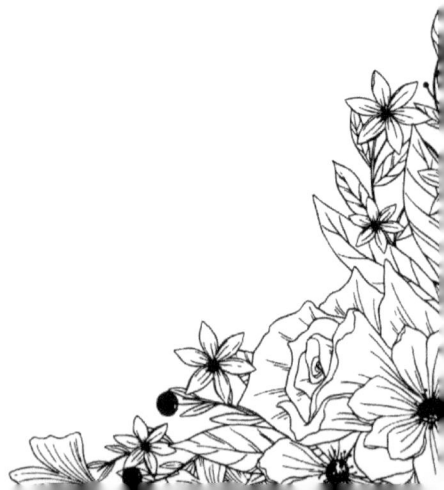

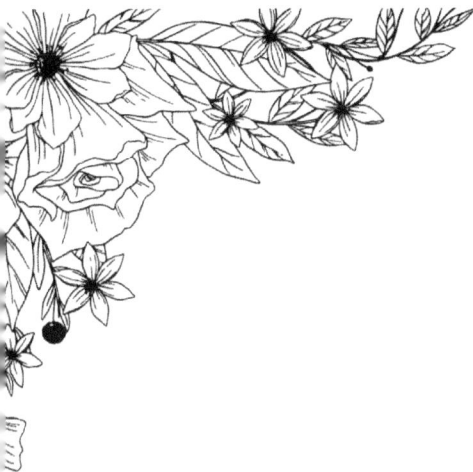

Forgive those who have committed an unforgivable act!

Forgiveness is for you, not for them.

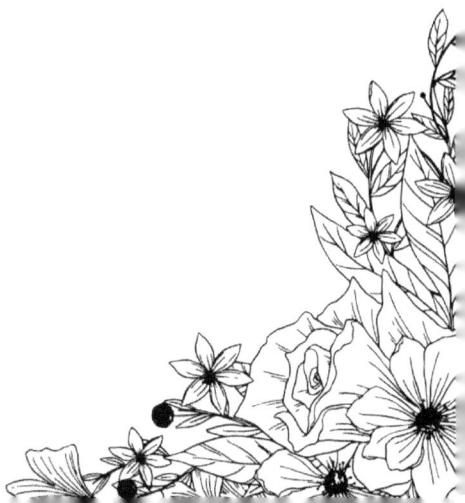

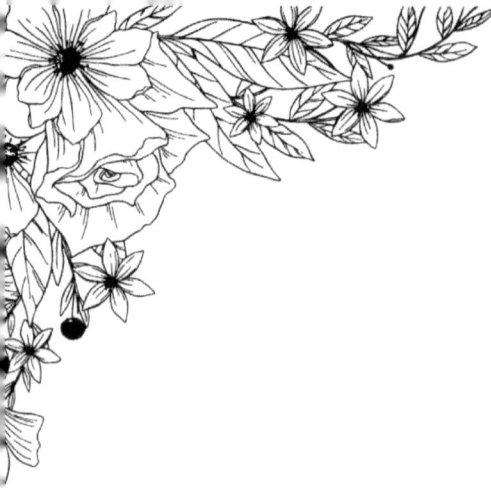

Stop recycling hurt!

Please.

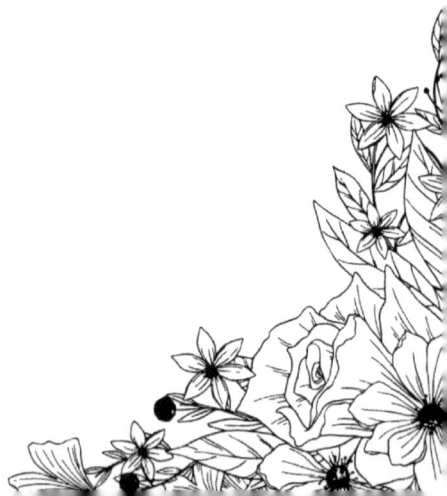

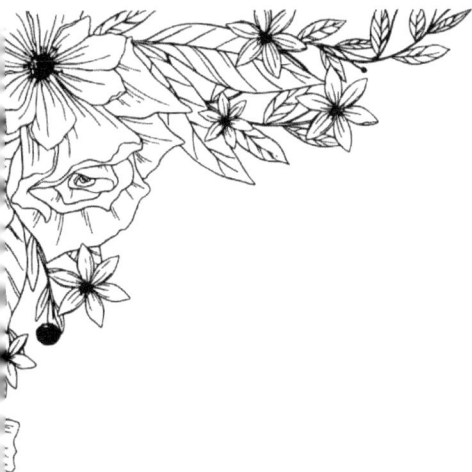

The body heals itself, but your mind and soul will
need your help with the healing process.

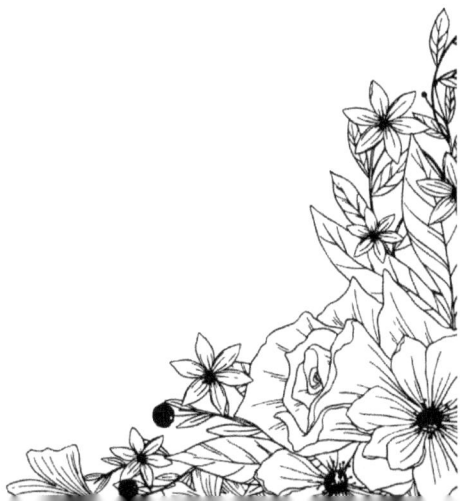

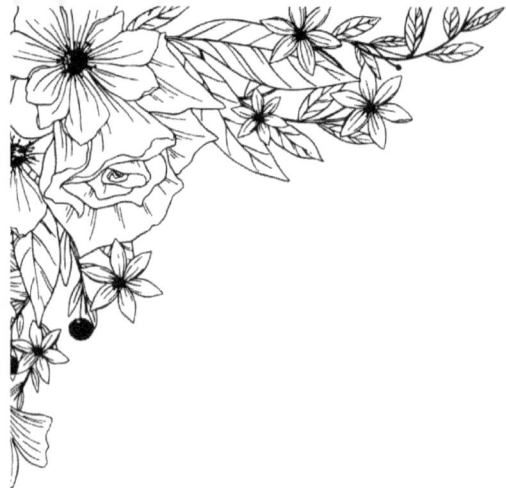

My bright smile did not always match how I felt on the inside. I am so glad I no longer have to fake it because I have finally made it. I am where I never thought I would be, in the land of contentment and peace.

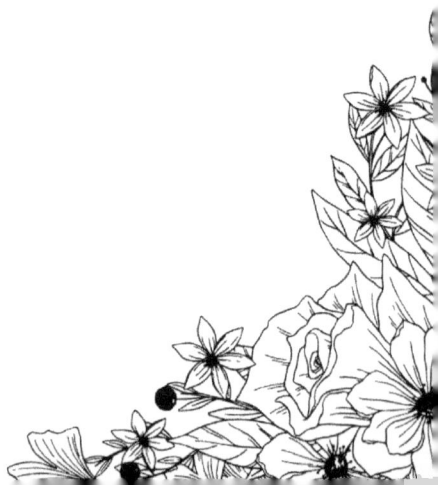

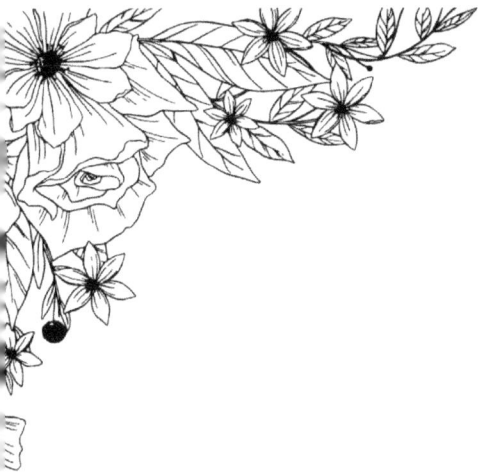

You cannot give birth to love when you are
pregnant with hate!

Release it.

You are only hurting yourself.

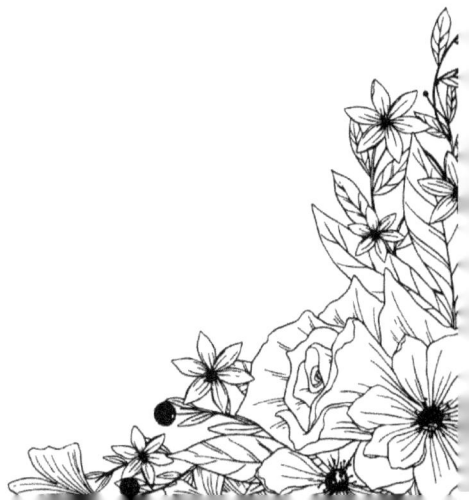

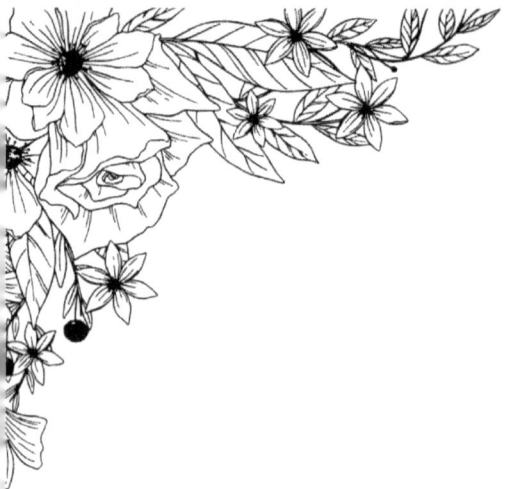

It is so easy to be bossy and lazy.

However, being a leader takes work.

It is so easy to be heartbroken and sad.

However, healing takes work.

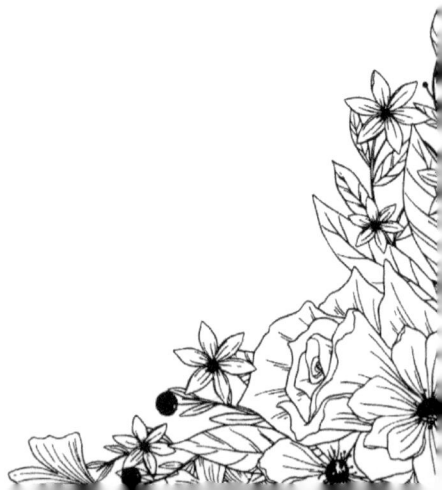

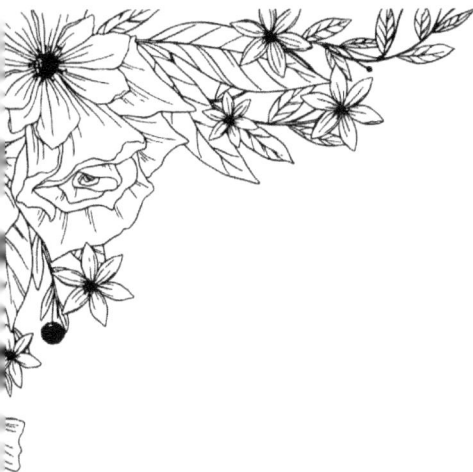

When you want to run back to a person because you "miss" them, take a moment and remember the bad! Chances are this person has not changed. The more you give to them, the more they are going to take, leaving you completely empty. If you want to miss someone, miss yourself. Miss the person you were before them and go get THAT person back.

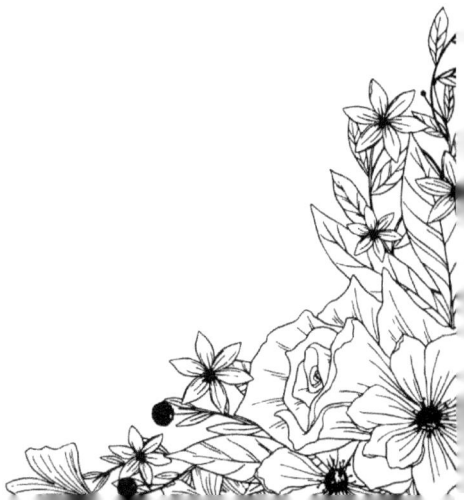

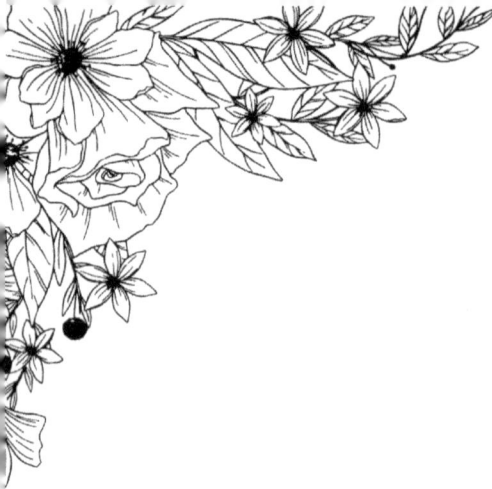

Life has taught me that you cannot give unlimited chances for people to hurt you, because they will take every single chance you give.

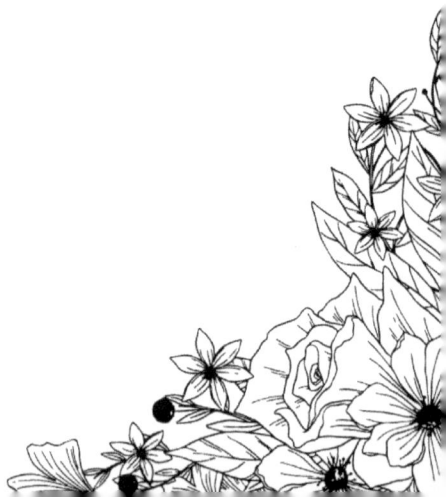

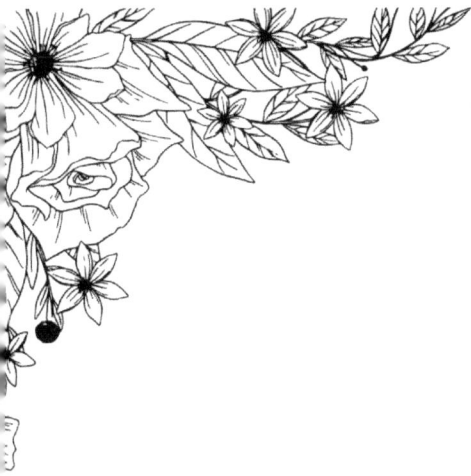

It is what you do in your valleys that will determine
how the view from your mountains will look.

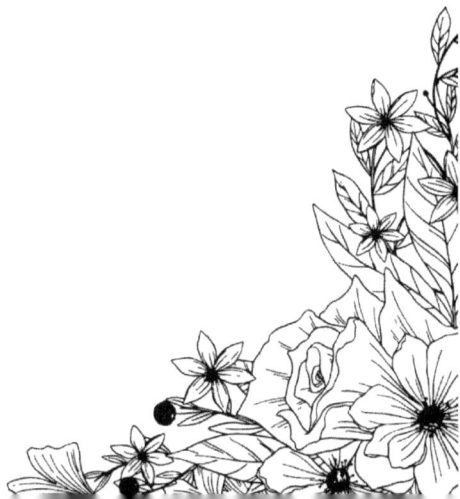

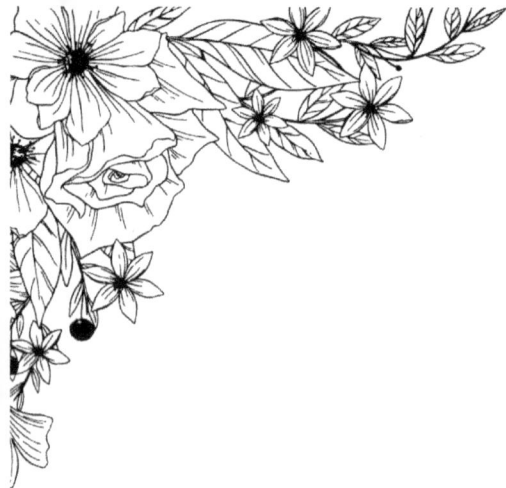

The thing I love most about self-love is that when I wake up in the morning, I know it will still be there.

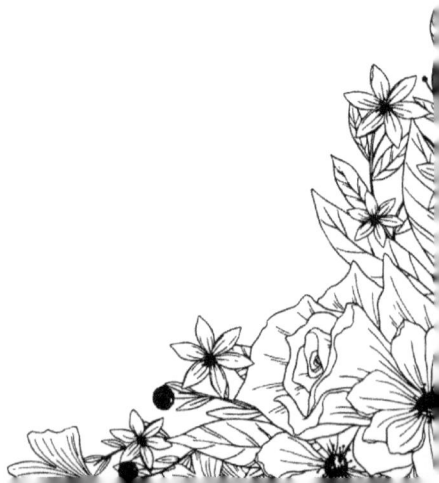

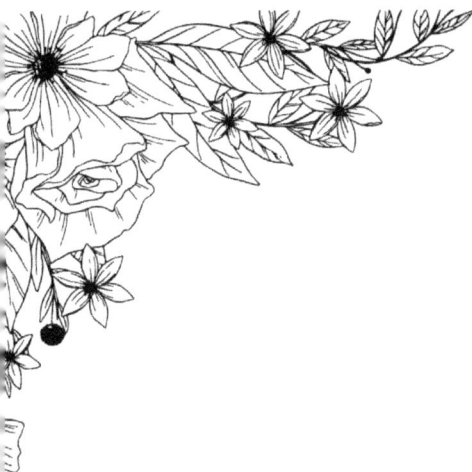

I used to do everything I could to get others to see me as a person who was valuable. I failed to realize the only person I had to convince was myself.

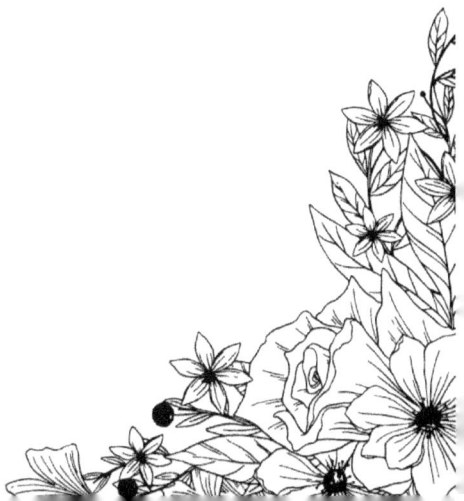

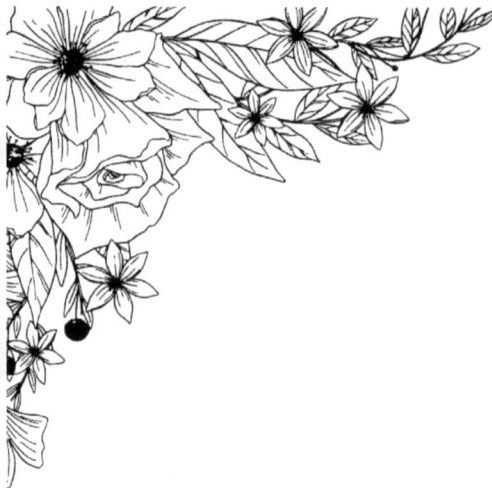

Honesty Time: Yes, sometimes I miss my ex, and I want to reach out to him, but I know nothing will come from that decision, but disappointment and regret. I believe self-love is when you sacrifice what you want for what you know you truly need.

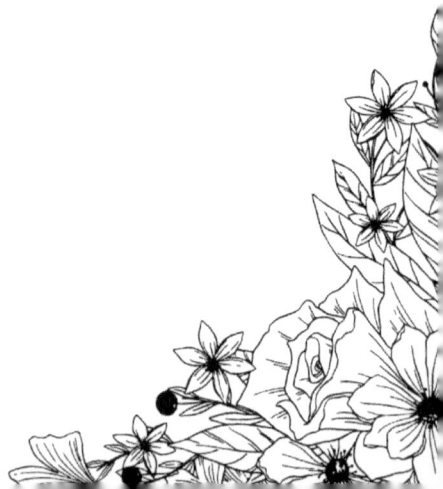

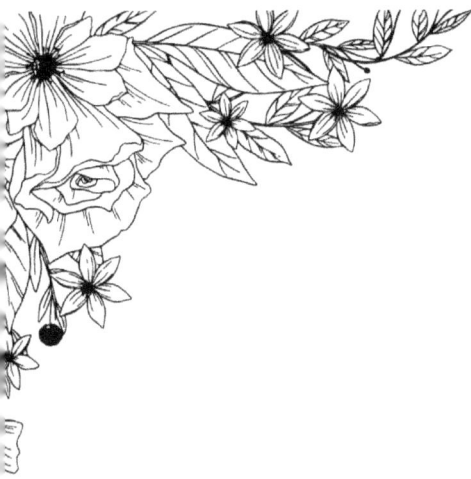

## One. Day. At. A. Time!

We are only given one day at a time because that is all we can handle. Live in this day. Love this day. Bask in this day. Be thankful for this day because someone, somewhere, did not get a chance to see it. May we always be grateful for the small things we often take for granted.

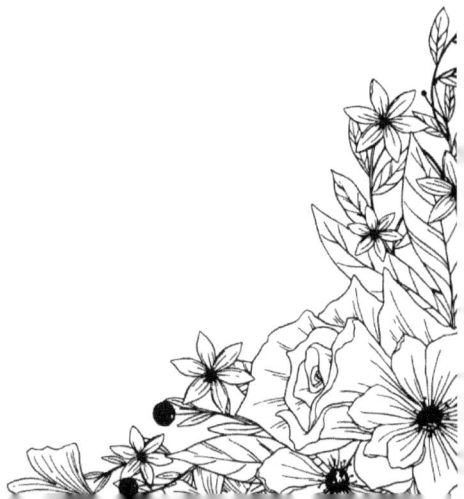

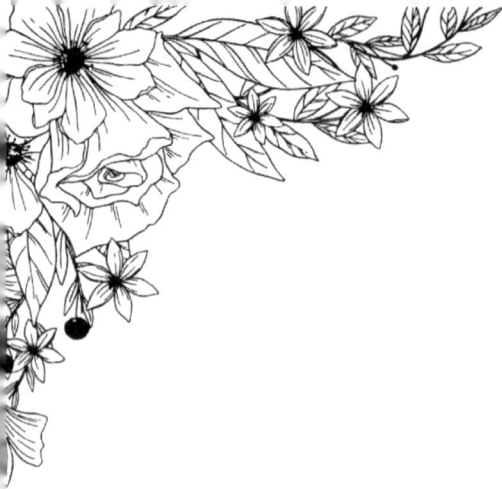

The stakes are too high to keep taking chances with
your emotions.

It is not worth it.

Protect yourself.

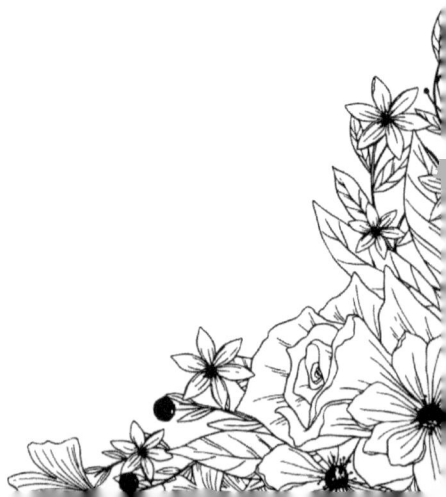

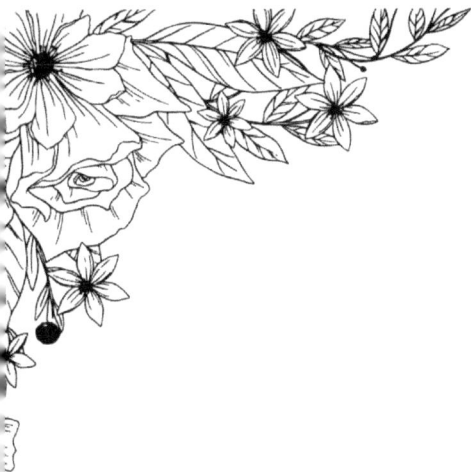

You cannot expect everyone to love the same way you love. You will end up disappointed every single time.

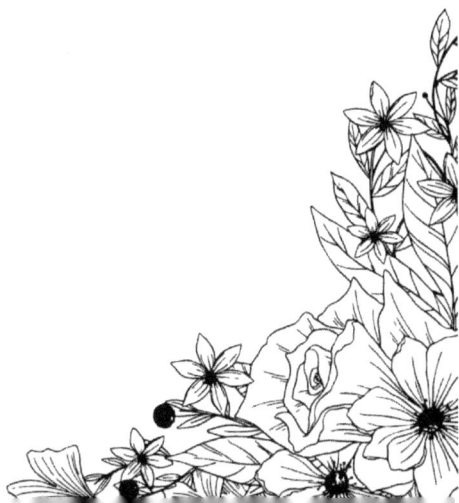

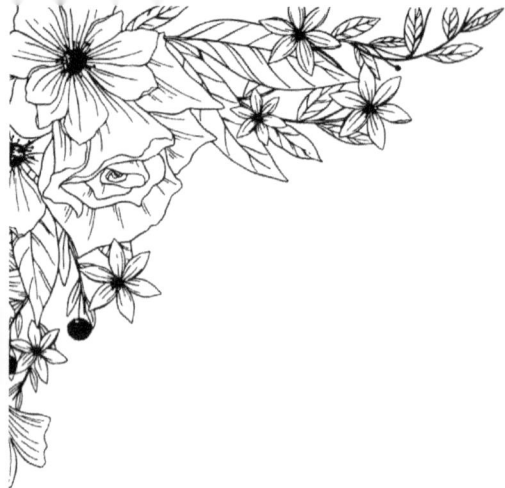

A person who does not have feelings will always tell you that you are "in yours". Do not listen to them. You were born to feel!

Feel. Completely.

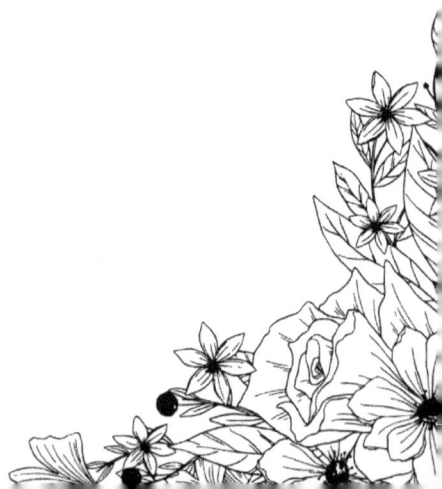

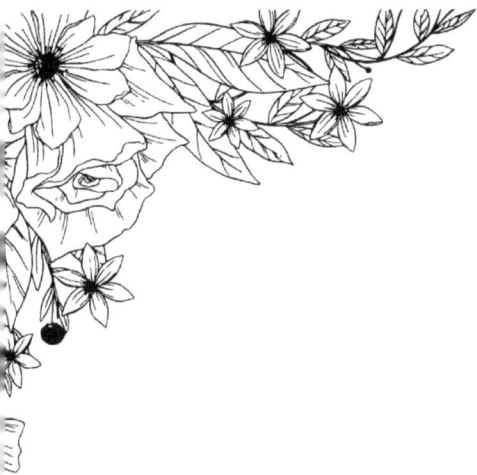

Stop looking to broken people for the answer on
how to fix yourself.

They do not have it.

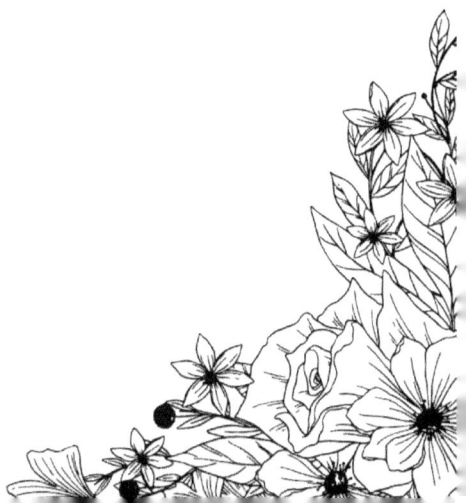

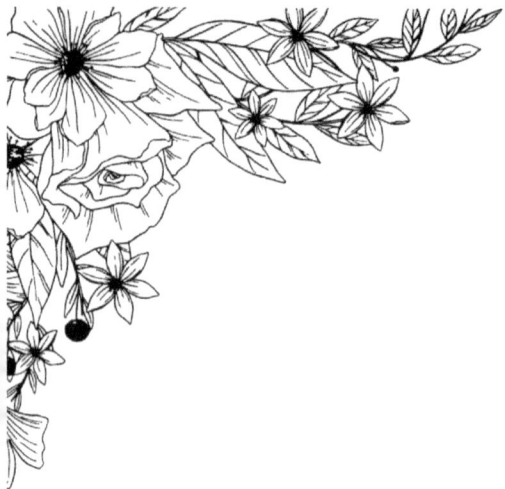

Stop auditioning for roles you were literally born to play.

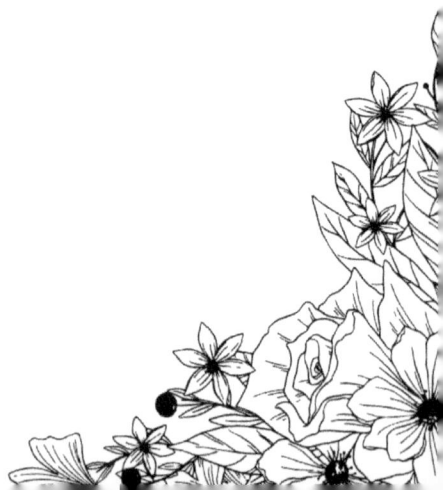

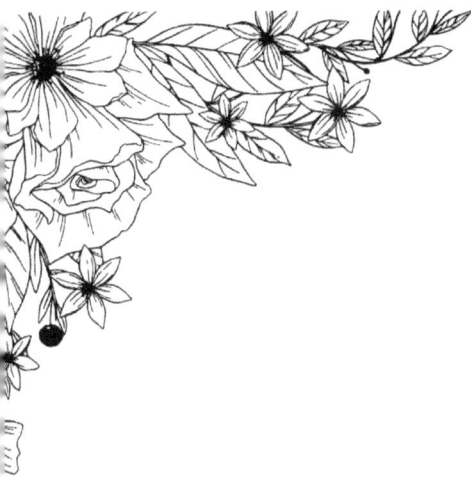

Stop trying to prove your worth to someone.

The right person will already know what you are worth when they meet you.

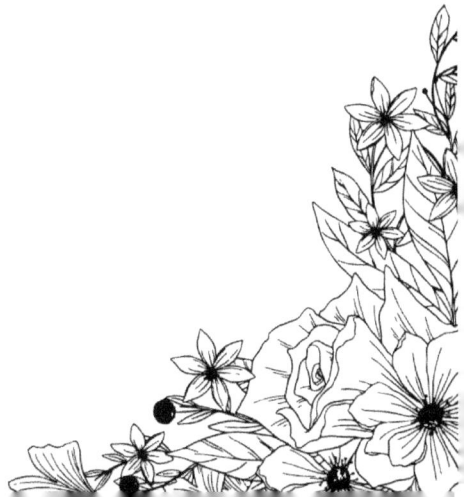

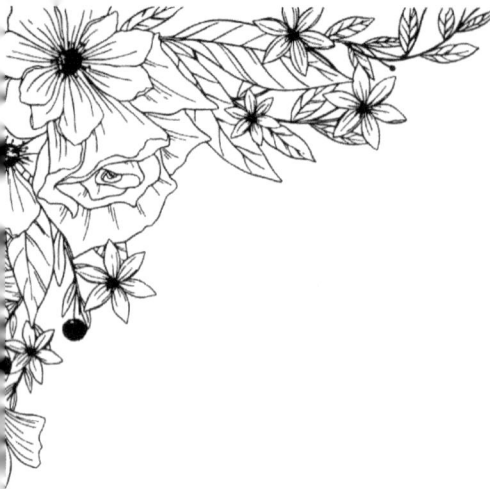

Trying to love a selfish person is like pouring your favorite drink into a cup with a big hole in it.

The cup will always remain empty.

Stop pouring yourself into someone who has "holes" in them, or you will always remain empty!

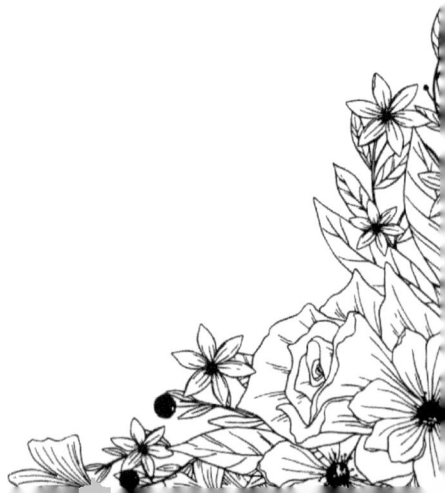

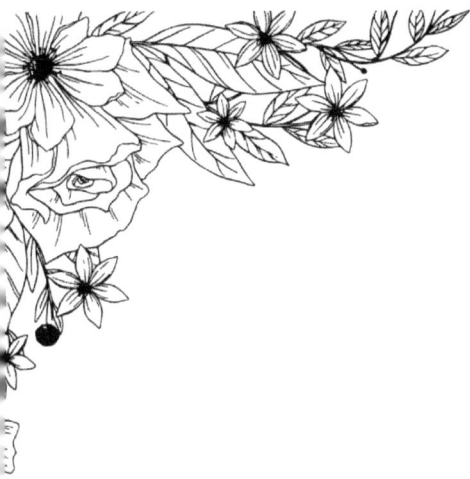

The pain you felt.

The hurt you experienced.

It does not even begin to compare to the love you
will receive.

But first, you must give that love to yourself.

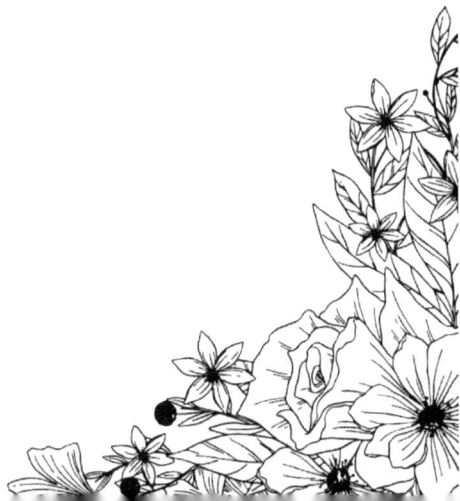

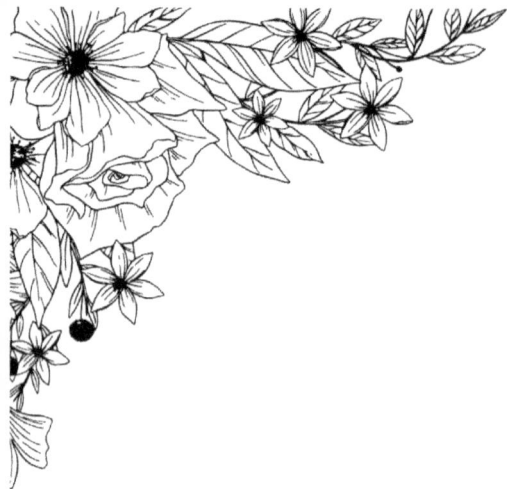

I never imagined being content in singleness, but each day I find myself. I have to say, I love who I have found. I did not know I was lost, but the truth is I was lost. Lost in all the people I was once with. Many people do not know the significance of being with a person who uplifts you and truly loves you. When you are around someone who only destroys you, you begin to think that is all you deserve. Take your happiness back.

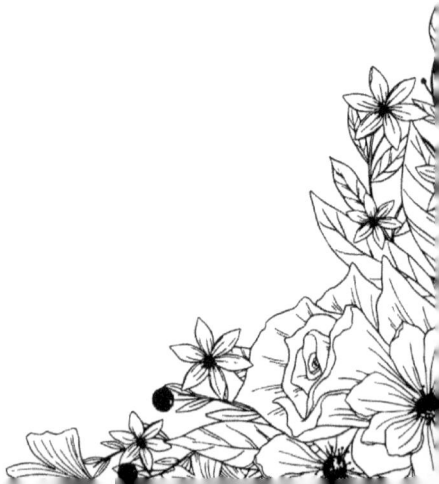

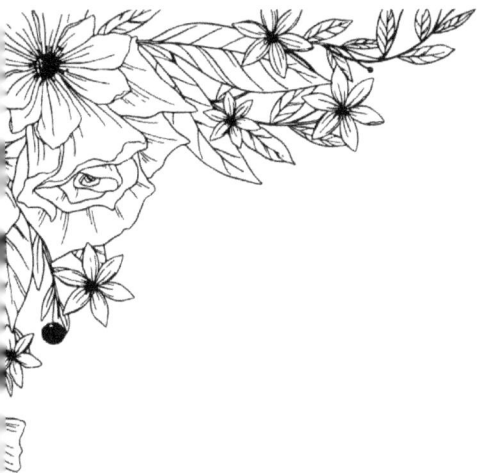

She was expected to be everything to everyone else, but when it came to her, nobody was there for her.

So, she decided to be everything to herself and let everybody else go.

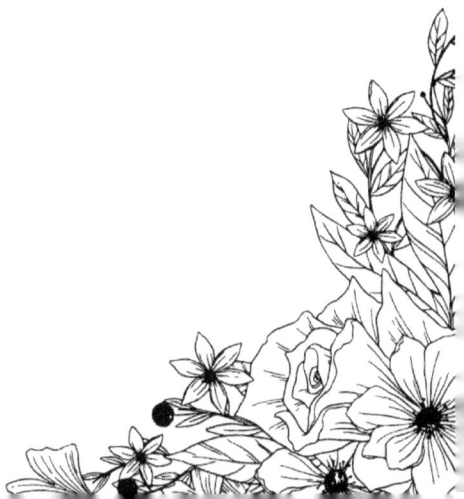

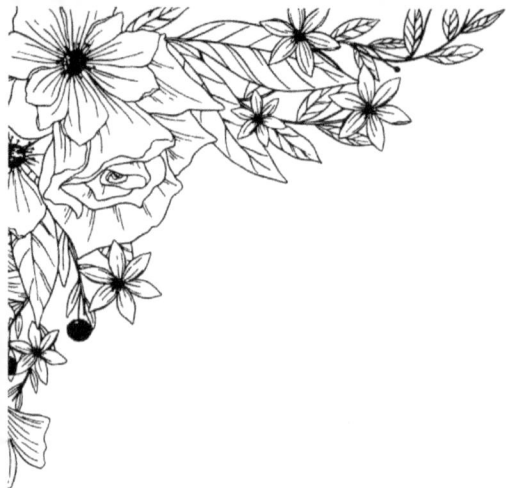

Daily Reminder: You need no one's permission to love yourself!

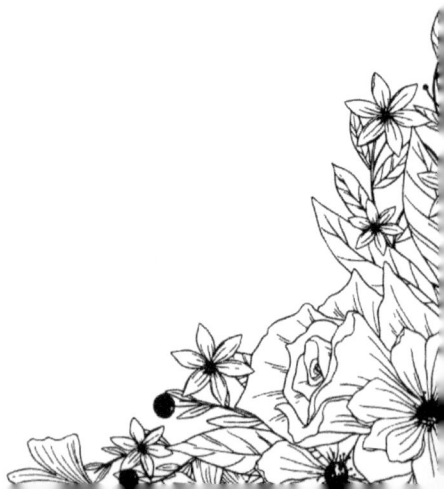

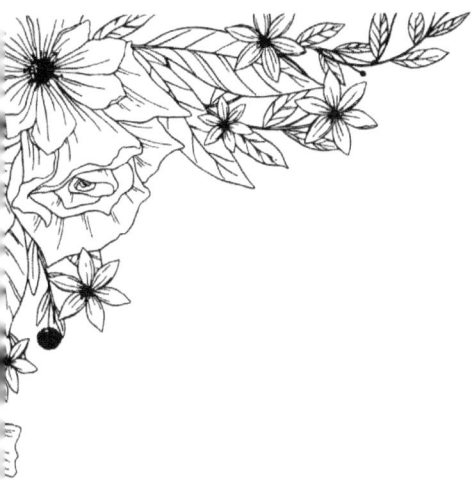

Your main responsibility in life is to make sure you are okay, every day. That is your one job.

Are you clocking in today?

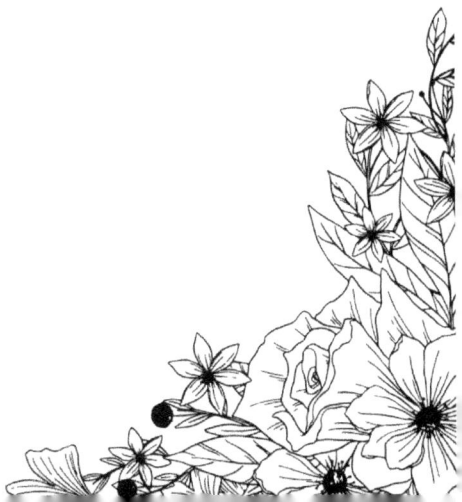

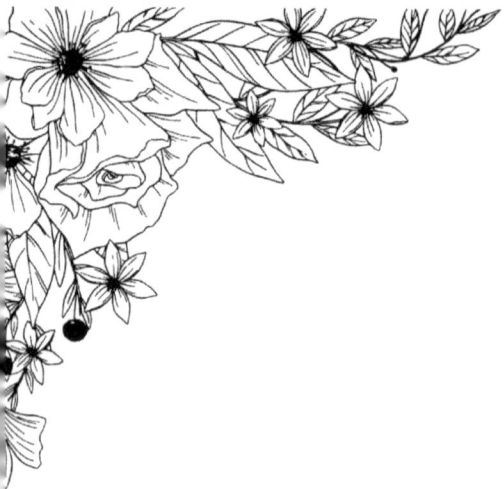

One should be more worried about losing themselves than losing someone they never truly had.

Take care of you.

Everyone else will just have to wait.

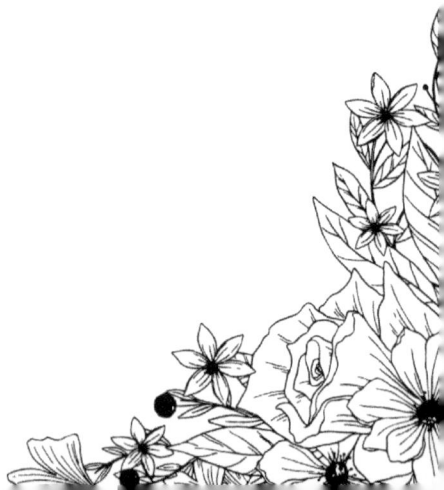

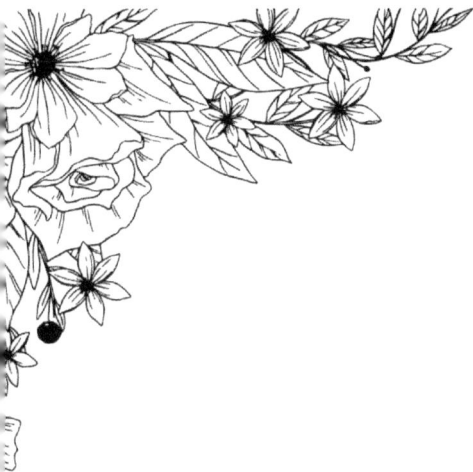

Your security is not the responsibility of someone else. Secure yourself! If someone comes along offering security, you will already have it, and you will not have to worry about them removing it when they feel like it.

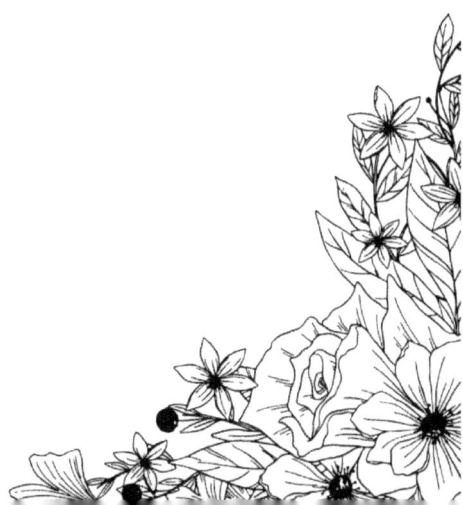

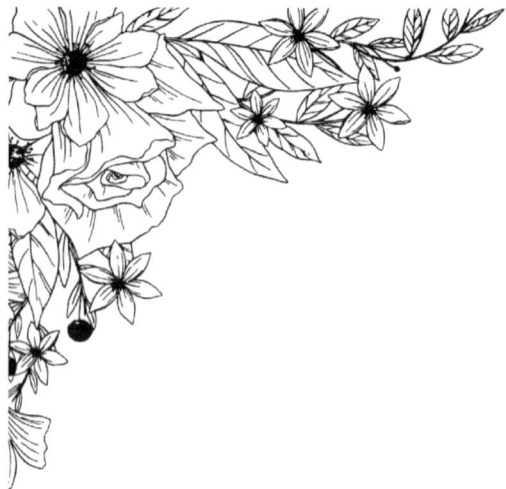

When you feel like you need a break, take it. It is your life. You do not have to explain why you are doing what is best for you.

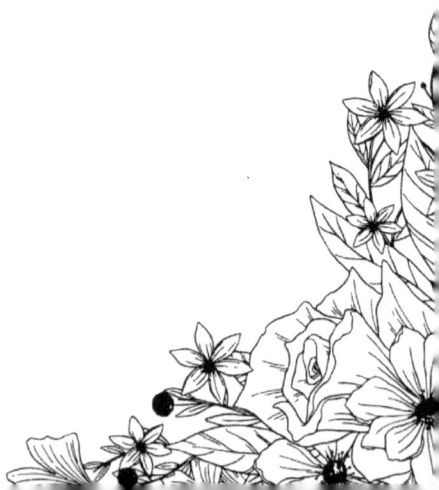

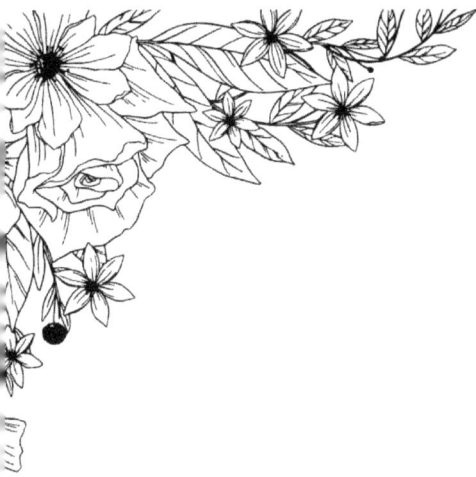

Daily Reminder: Inhale Love. Exhale Hate!

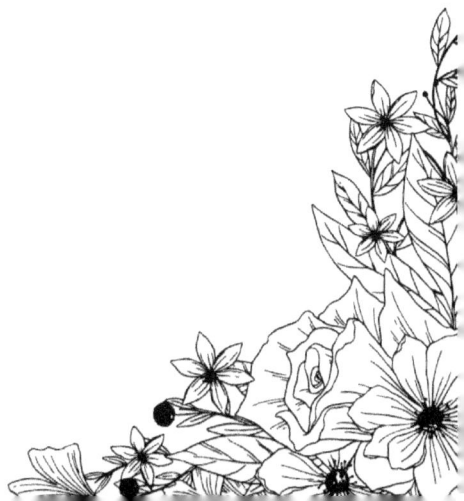

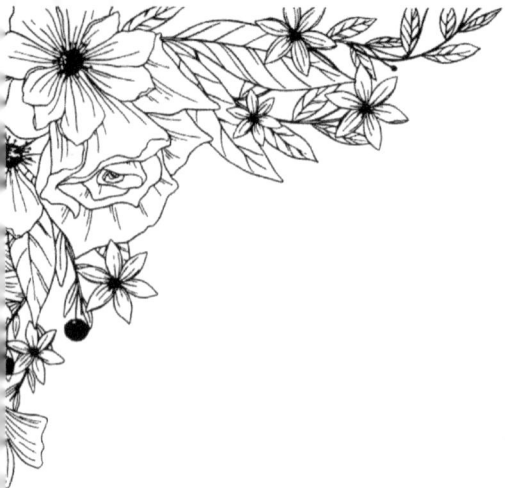

Loving myself gives me permission to be free, healthy, and aware of what I truly need. So, I am here to tell you, loving yourself is not VANITY. It is SANITY!

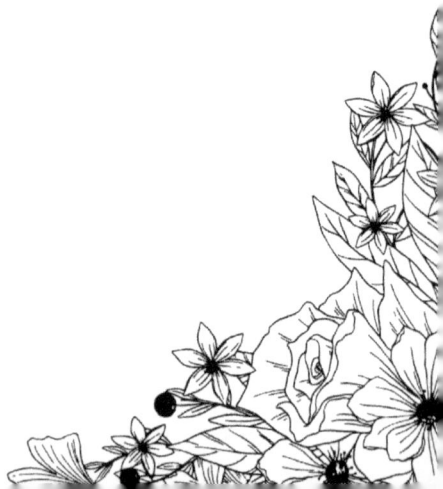

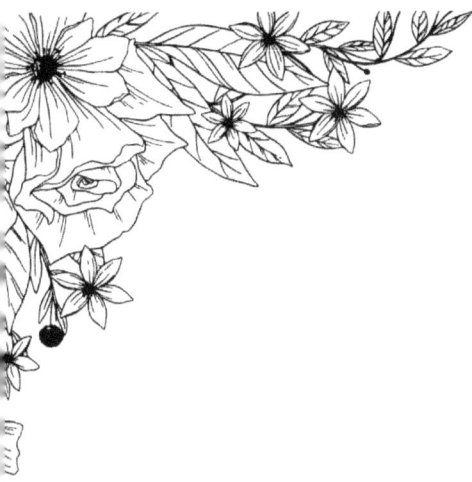

A person's inability to notice your worth does not
make you worthless!

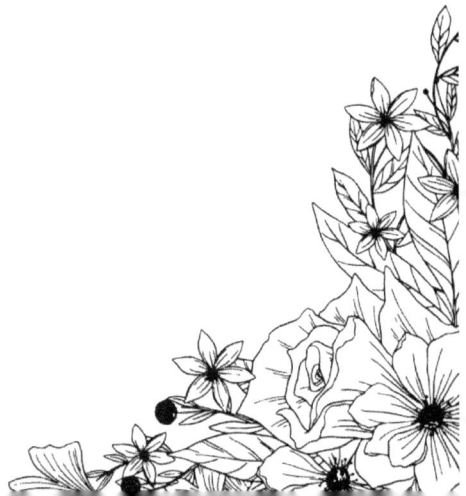

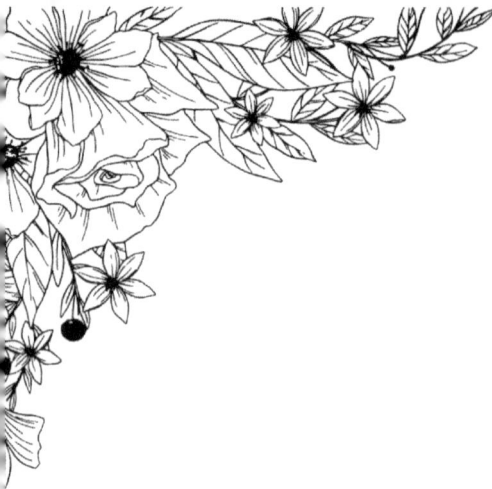

Do not wait for people to show you that you are an option to them before you decide to make yourself a priority.

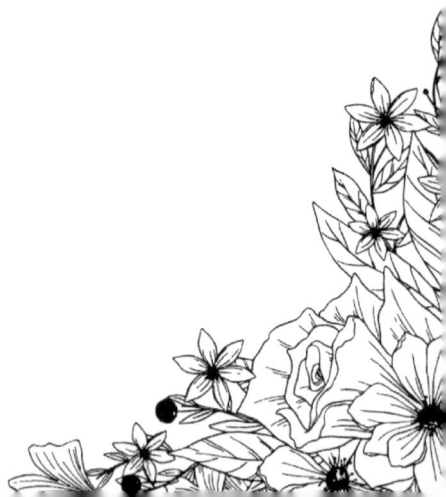

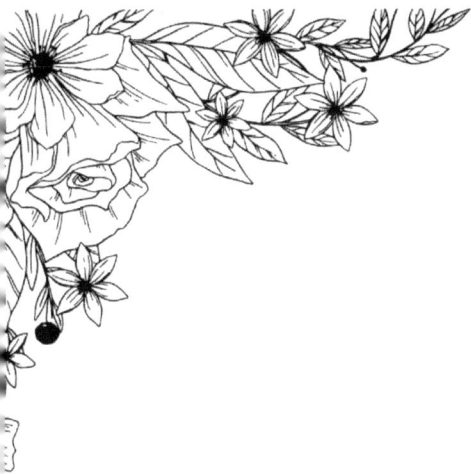

Daily Reminder: At the end of the day, you are all you have. Be good to you.

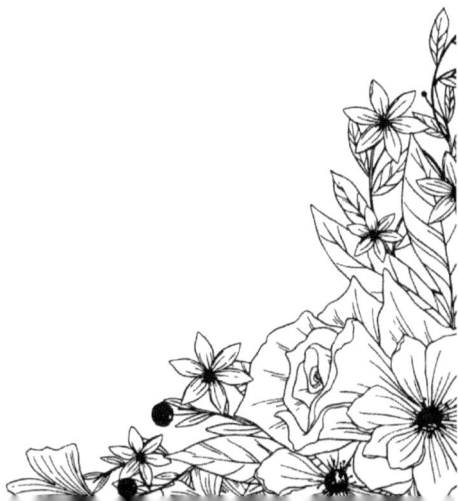

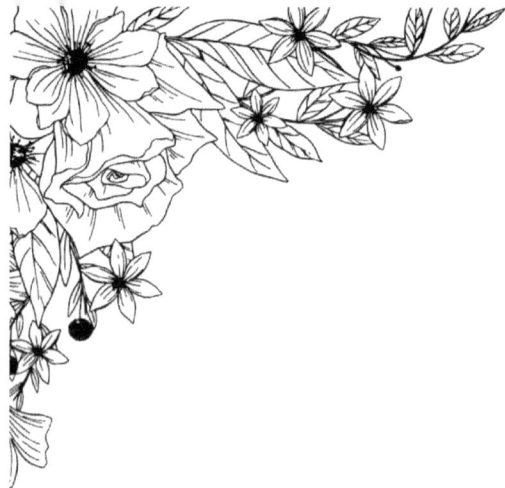

Being single is not a time to go looking for someone to be in a relationship with. It is the time to discover who you are as an individual.

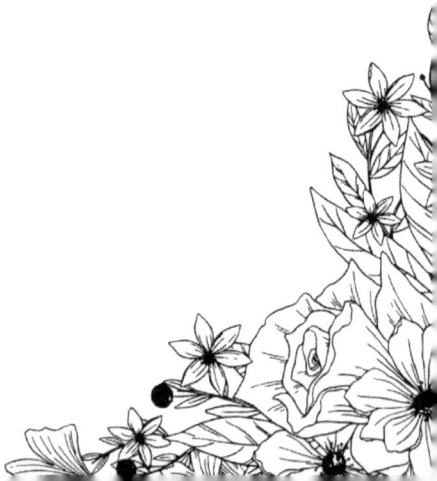

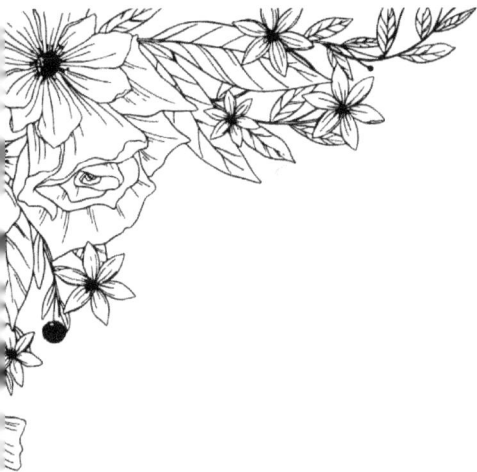

Daily Reminder: Mistakes are proof that you are trying, so do not give up.

Keep trying.

Keep making mistakes.

Keep being great.

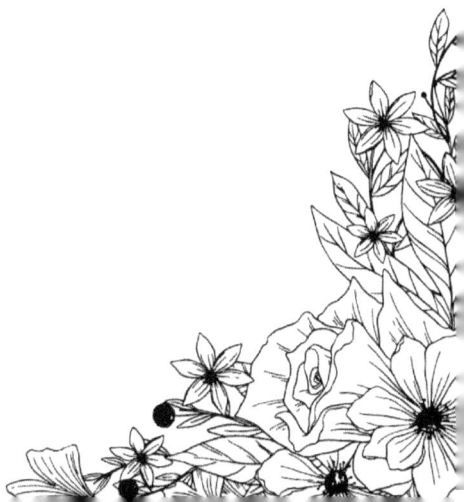

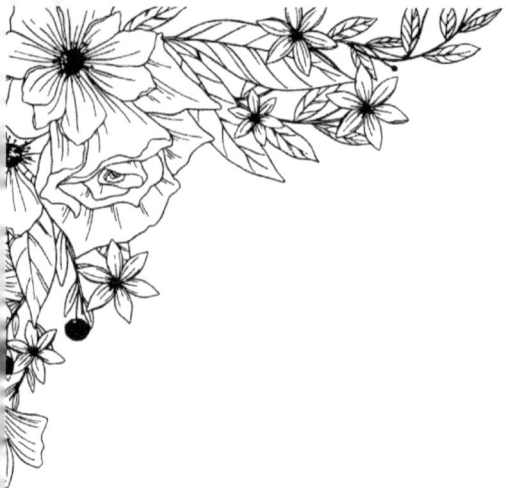

Daily Reminder: It is perfectly acceptable to heal and love again!

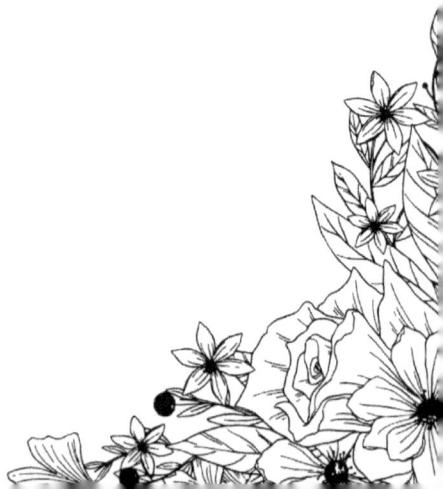

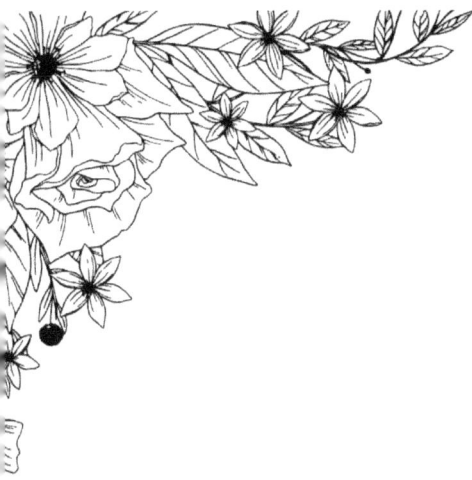

Daily Reminder: Despite popular opinion, it costs absolutely nothing to be kind!

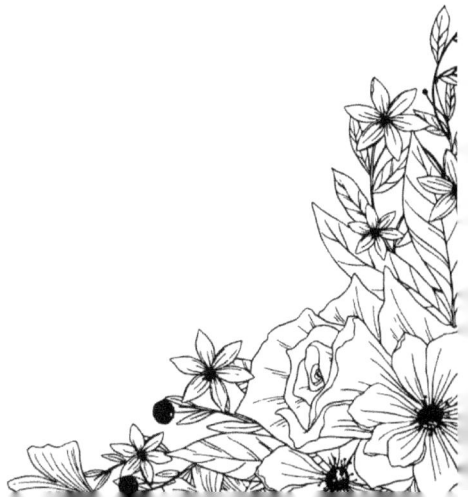

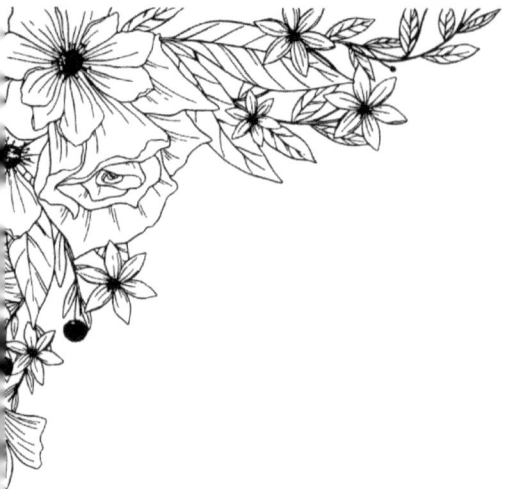

Daily Reminder: You made it through the last obstacle.

You will make it through this one!

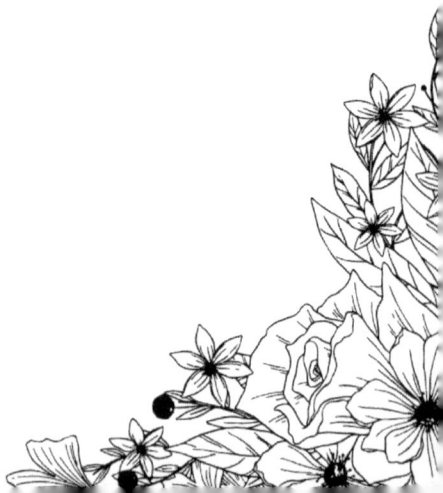

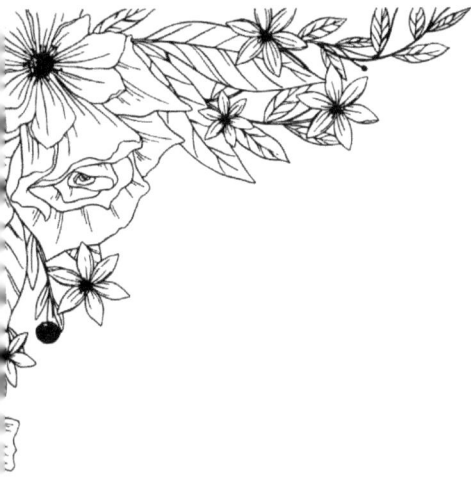

Live your life, not that you might prove others wrong, but that you might prove yourself right!

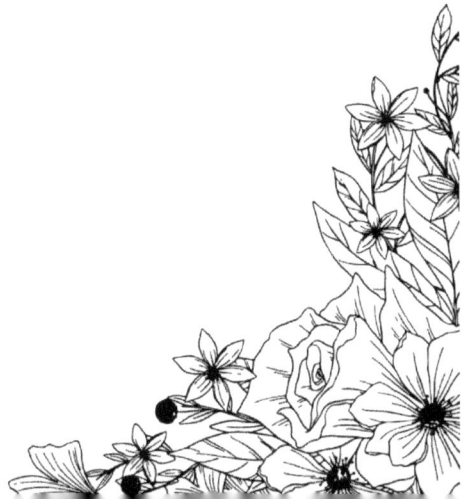

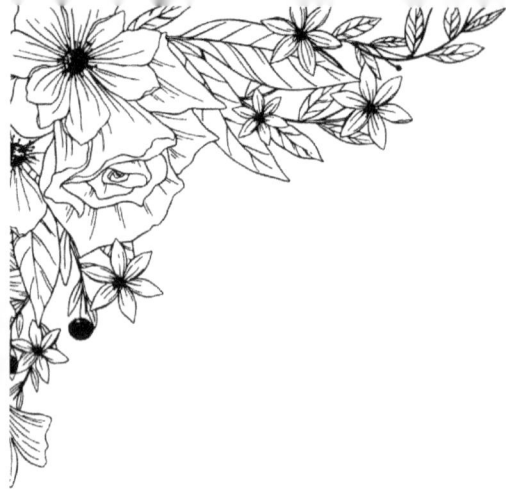

Daily Reminder: You made it through the last obstacle. You will make it through this one!

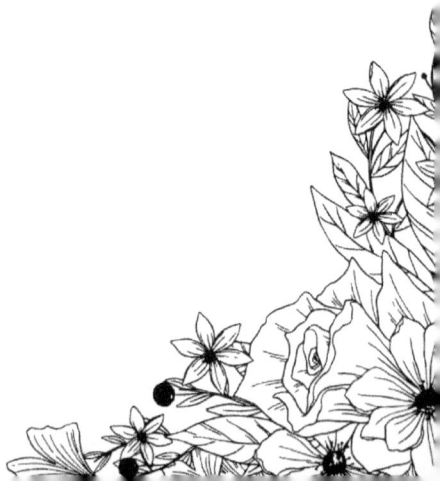

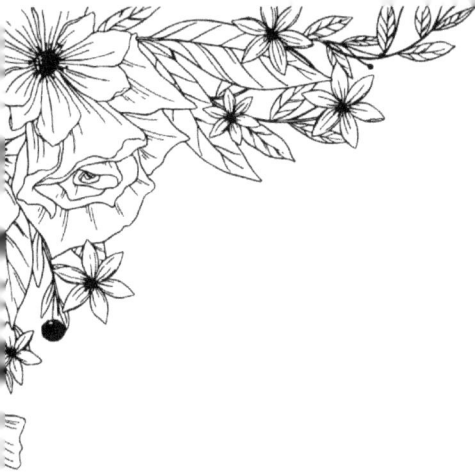

You are an island!

It is your choice whether you want company, or you want to be alone.

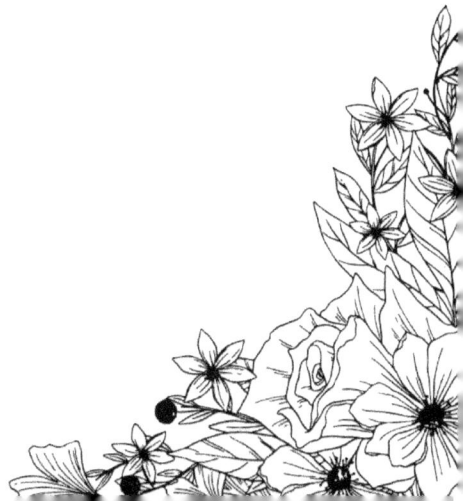

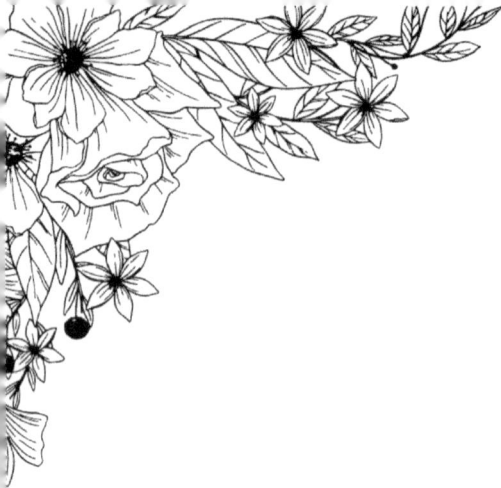

People who are bad for you will only see the bad in you.

People who are good for you will only see the good in you.

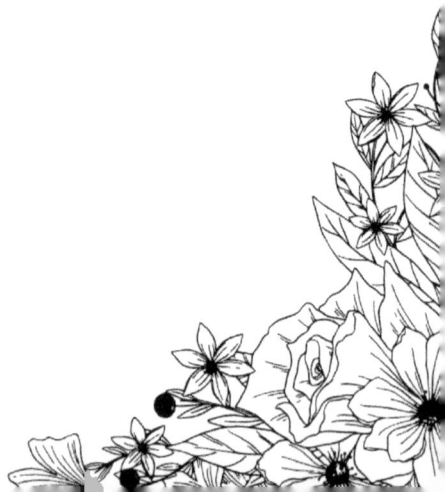

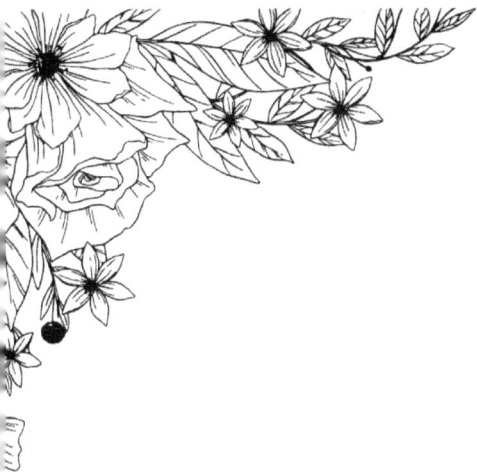

As the sun rises from the water and shines on the trees, it signals a new day.

It signals a new opportunity to be the best version of yourself.

It signals hope that you can follow your dream.

It signals that love has another chance to find you.

In those dark times, remember to hold on to the sun... hold on to hope!

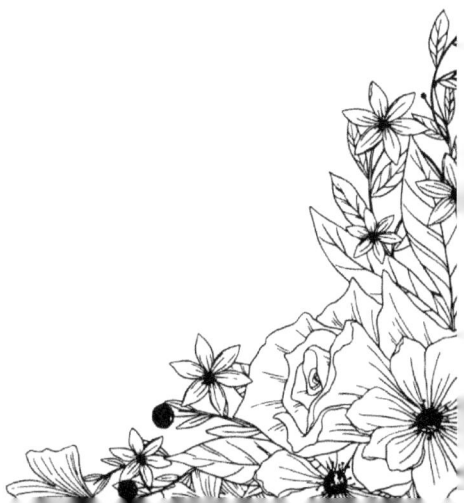

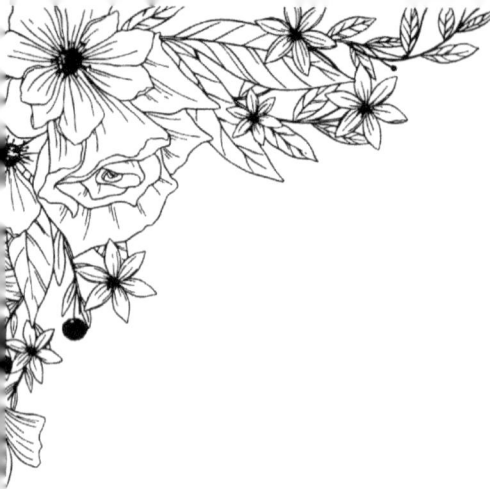

Do not allow others to make you feel crazy because you decided to take the necessary steps to better yourself.

Do what you need to do for you.

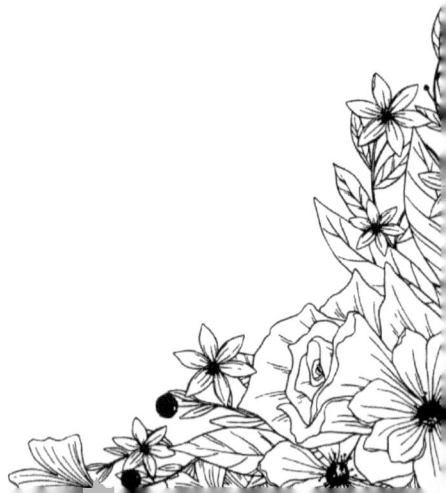

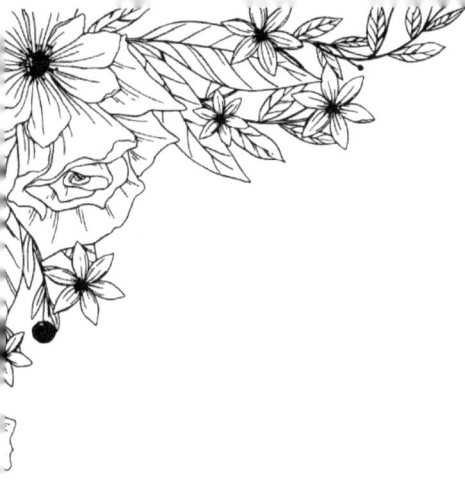

Friendly Reminder: God woke you up for a reason.
Find that reason and chase it until it is yours!

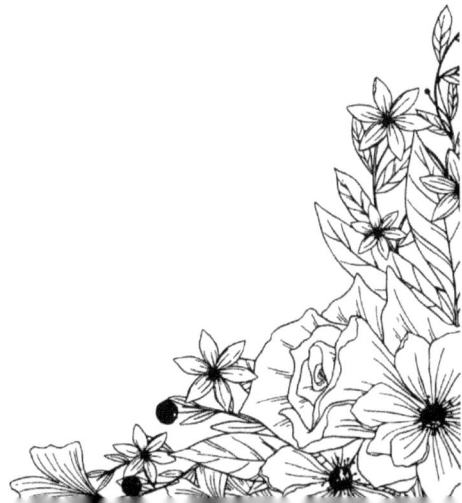

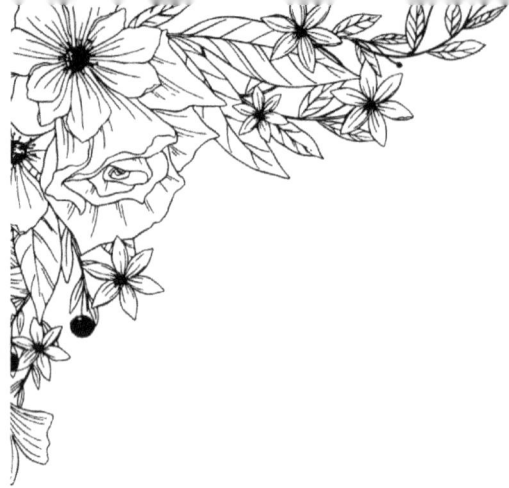

You owe no one an explanation for putting yourself first.

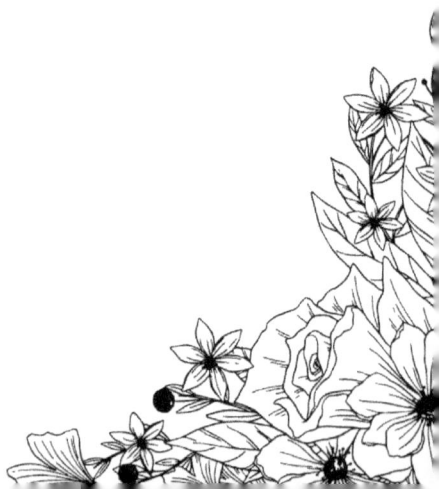

Love you!

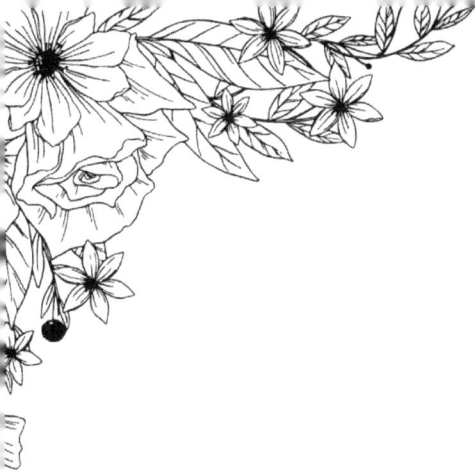

That is the least you can do.

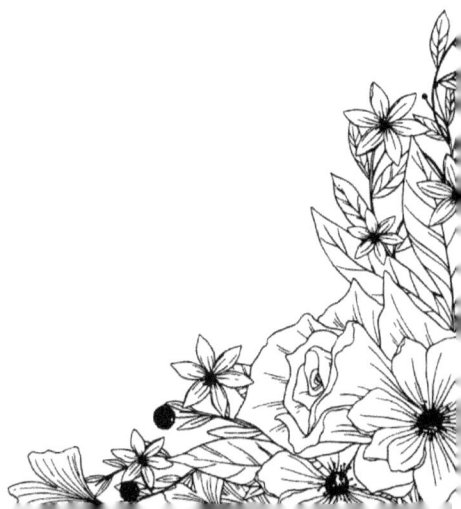

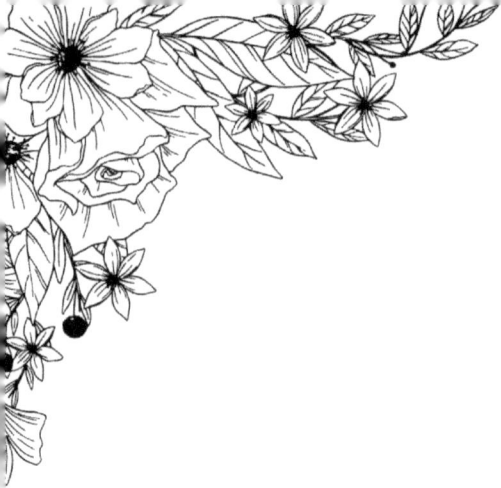

You do not get to put a timetable on my healing.
I will be healed when I am healed. If my progression
of healing offends you, then that is solely on you.

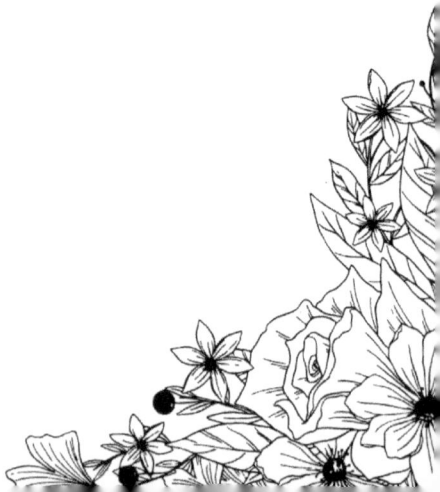

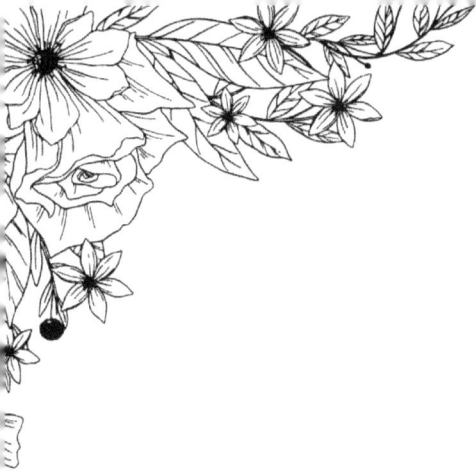

Gentle Reminder: It is perfectly okay to cry when you need to!

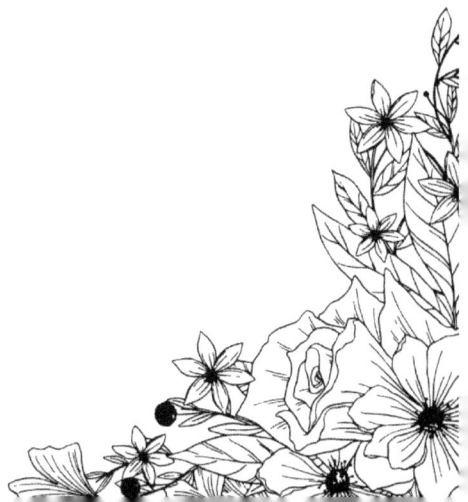

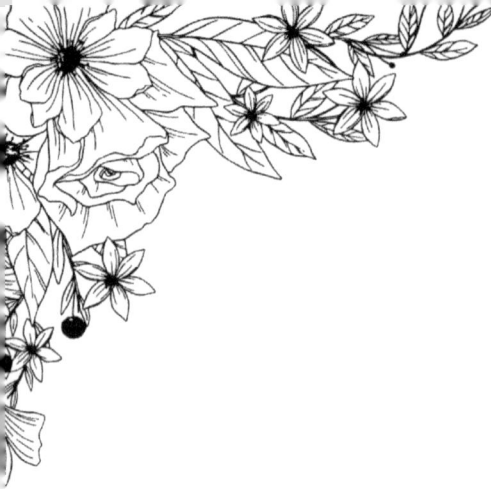

Love Yourself OR Lose Yourself.

Your choice.

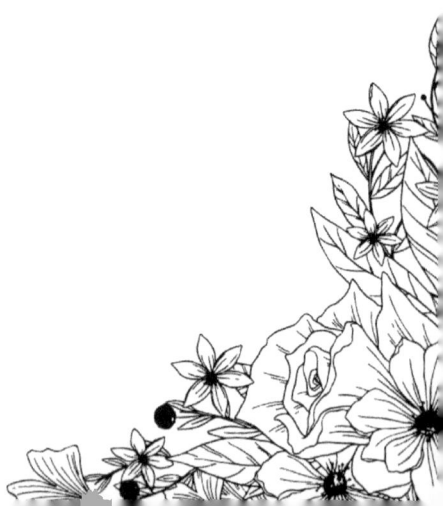

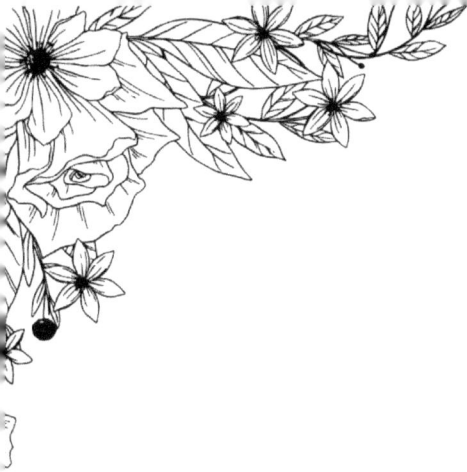

Take that break.

Cry those tears.

Share that emotion.

Speak your truth.

It is okay to be vulnerable and expressive.

It is okay to still be broken while you are healing.

Healing is a process, not a destination.

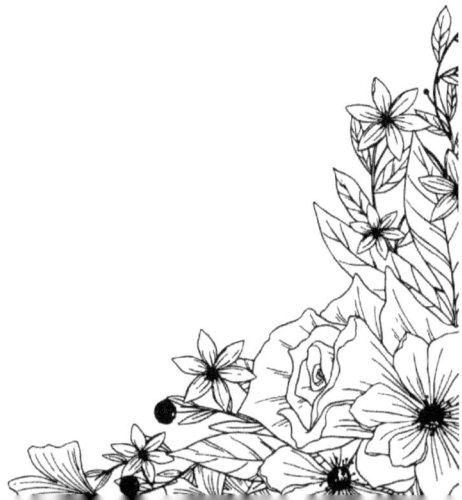

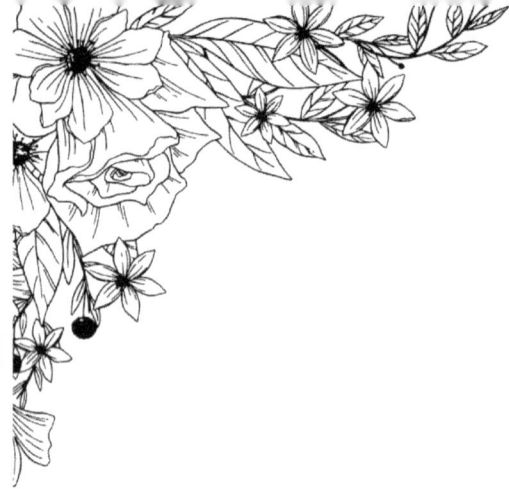

That which does not serve you, does not deserve you!

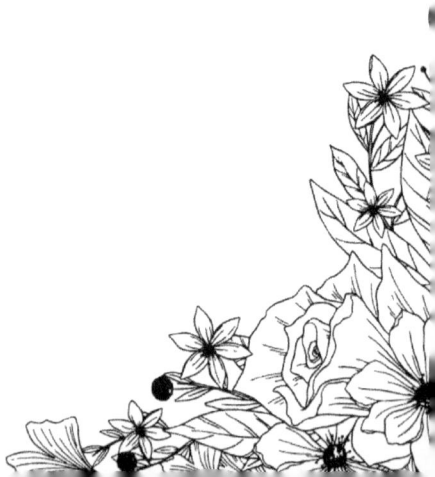

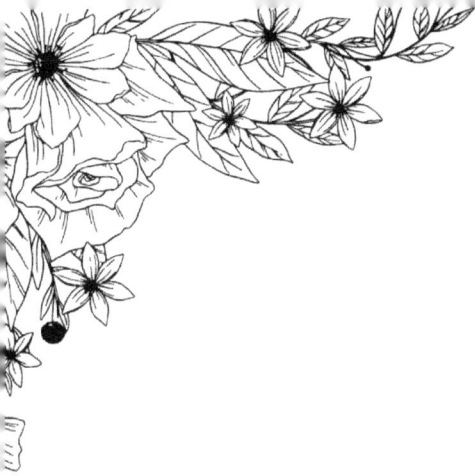

**BREAKING NEWS:**

Self-love does not equate to never desiring a relationship.

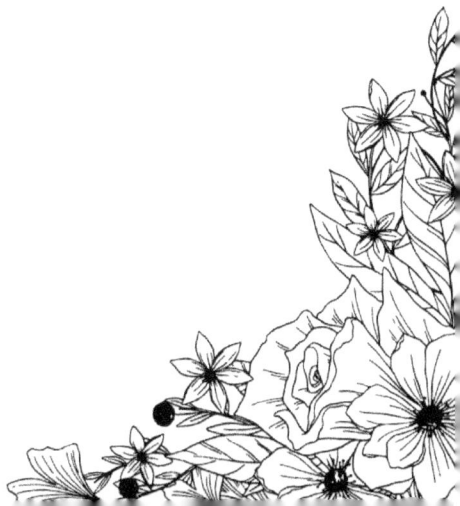

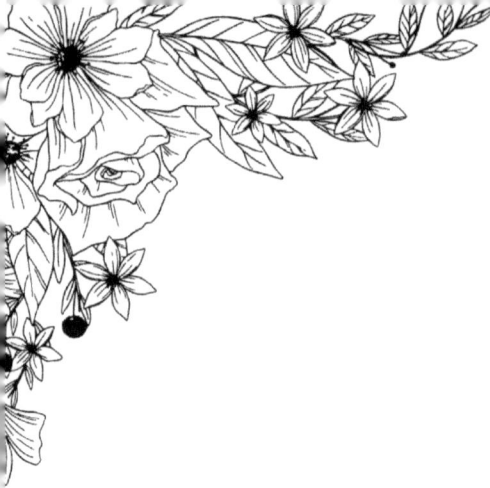

You are still magic!

Even on the days when you do not feel the most magical.

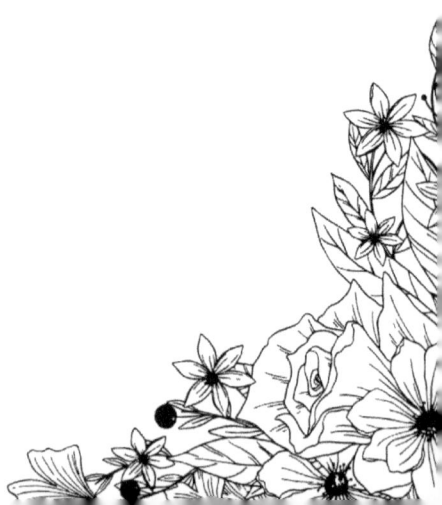

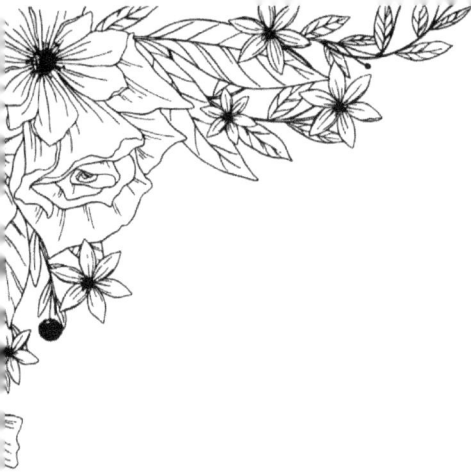

Stop discounting your heart and soul.

If someone cannot afford it, there is a reason.

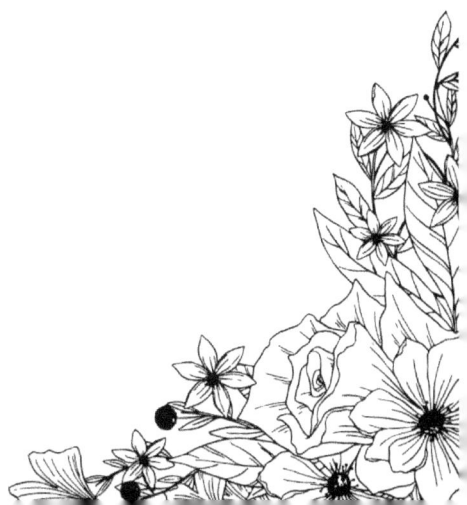

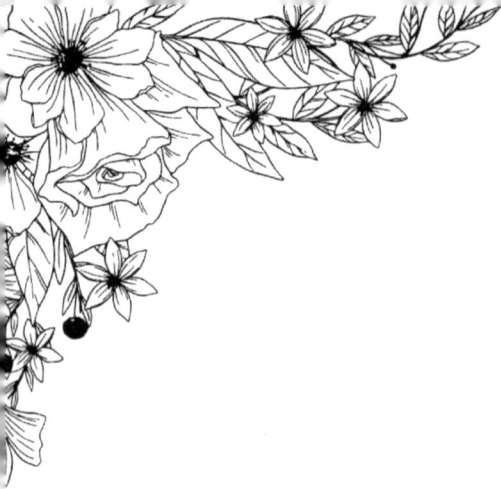

Sometimes the place that you are used to is not the place where you belong.

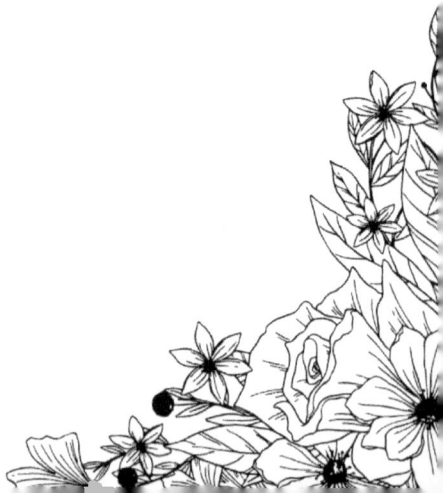

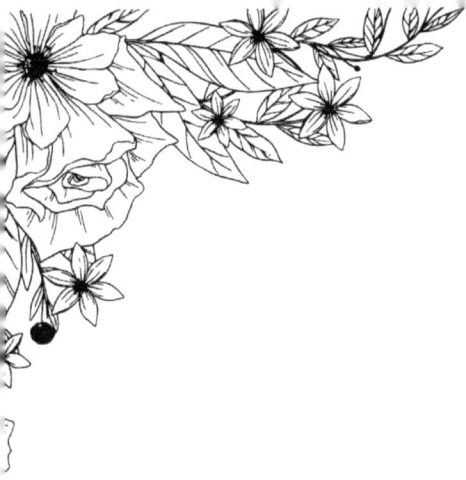

Once you realize that you do not like what a person is serving, excuse yourself from the table!

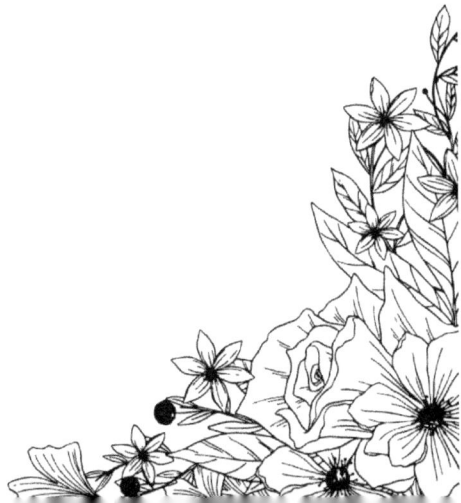

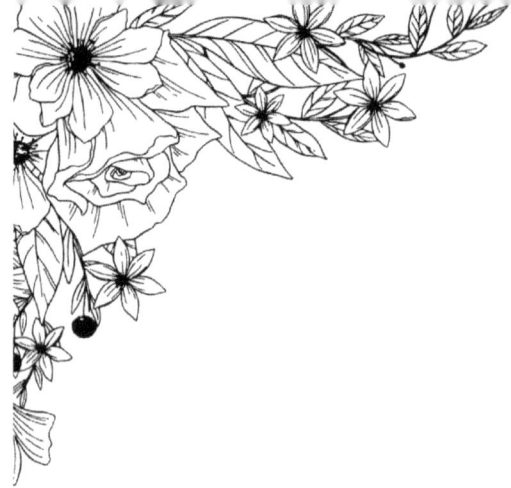

Pick your head up and stop mourning that past relationship!

You did not lose anything; you gained everything!

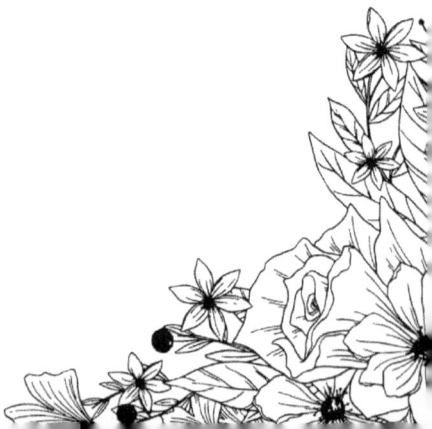

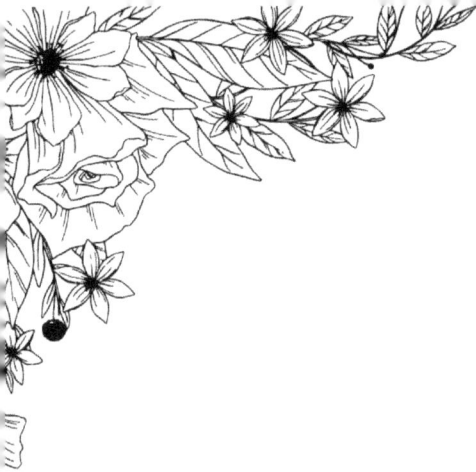

People will try to downplay and dismiss your progress because it may be going at a slower pace.

Answer me this though: Did not the turtle win the race?

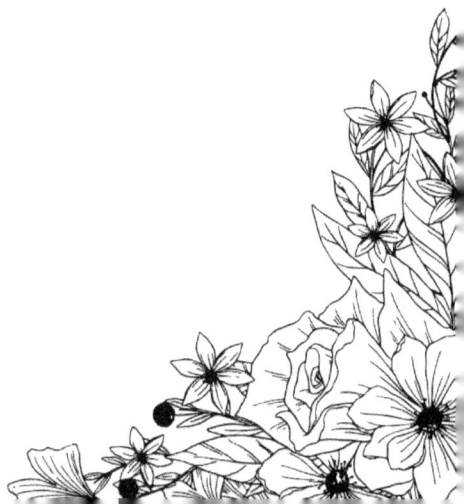

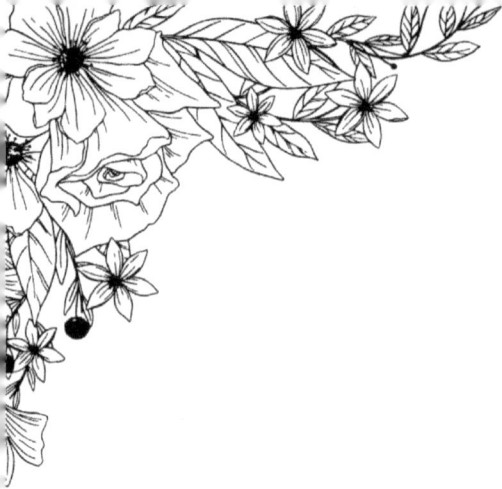

People will laugh at your standards when they have none!

Never change who you are.

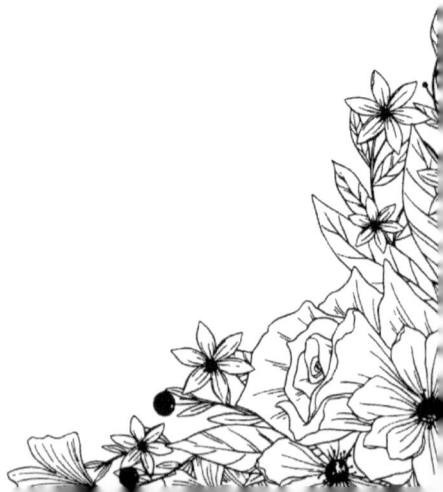

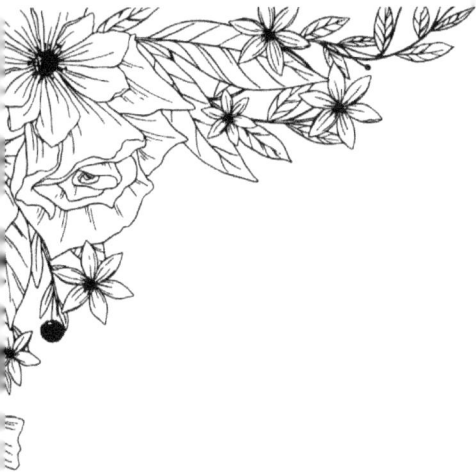

If you are everything to everyone else, what are you to yourself?

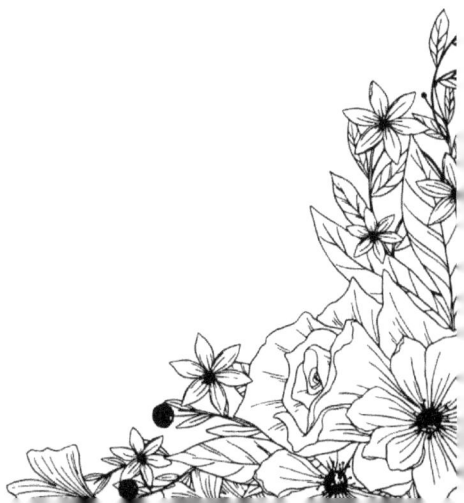

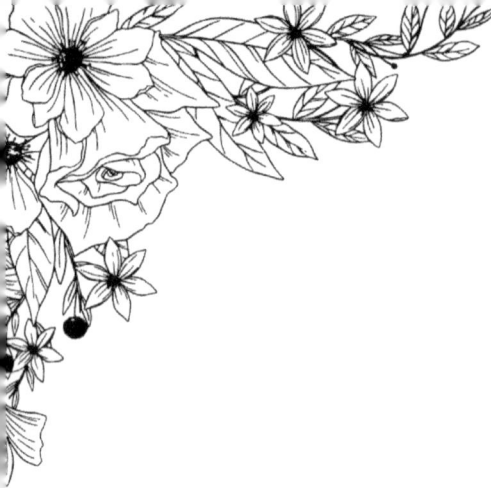

Stop minimizing your emotions and how you feel just so others may feel "comfortable"!

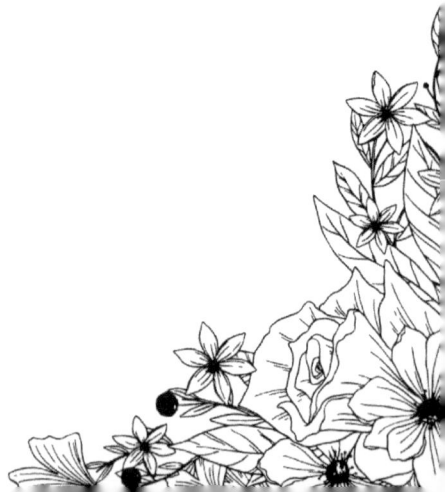

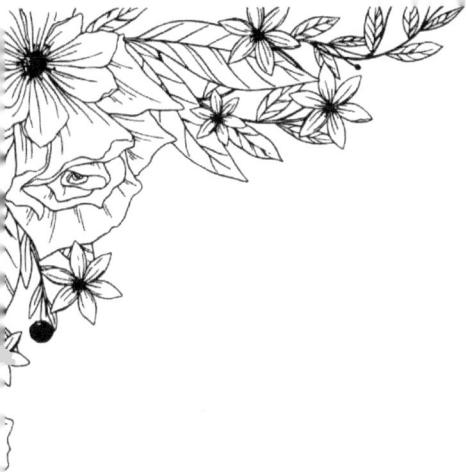

Focus on contentment not resentment.

Be happy with the life you have and let go of all the negativity that no longer matters!

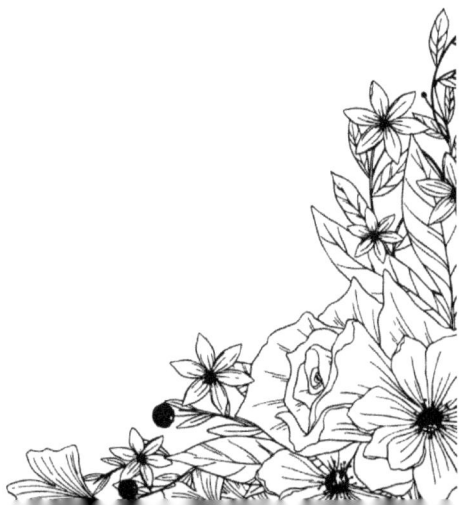

The best thing to do with your feelings is to feel them.

Do not push them down.

Do not dismiss them.

Do not downplay them!

FEEL THEM, DEEPLY!

And if you are around those who do not allow you to feel them, change the company you keep!

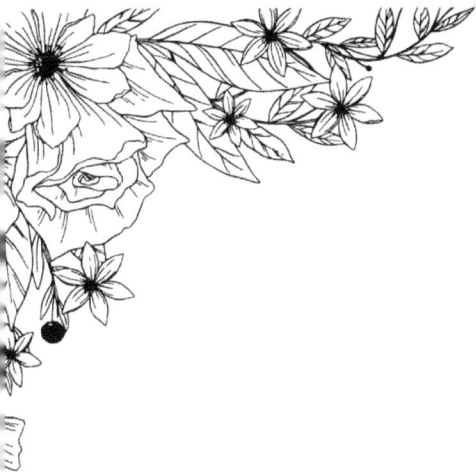

Someone's inability to see your greatness DOES NOT make you any less great!

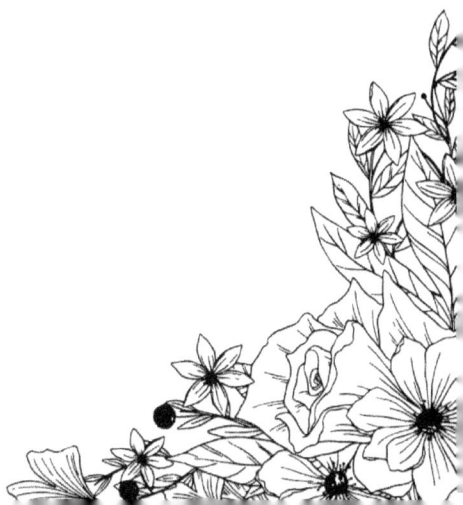

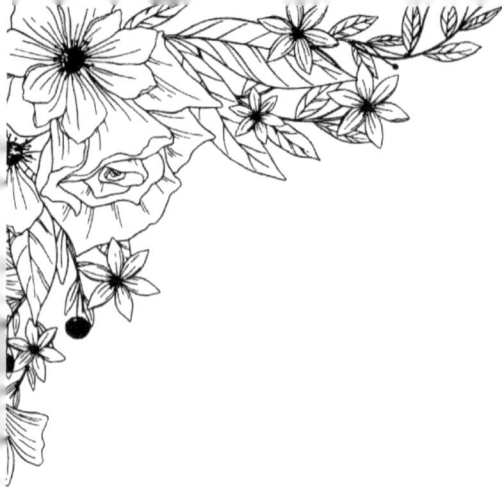

NEVER allow anyone to change you, unless you are a terrible person!

If you are unsure about the type of person you are, do some deep self-reflection.

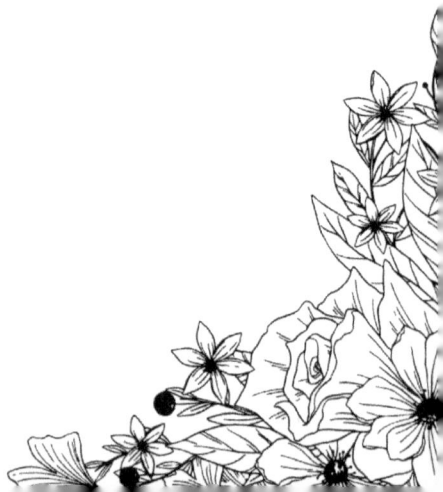

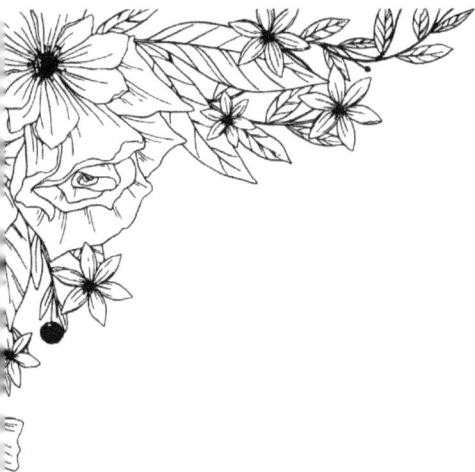

Today, and every day, be kind to yourself! You are trying. You are showing up. You are doing the best you can. You are enough! It is okay to show yourself some kindness!

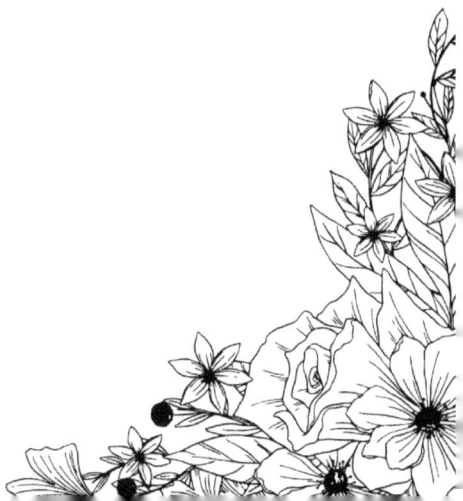

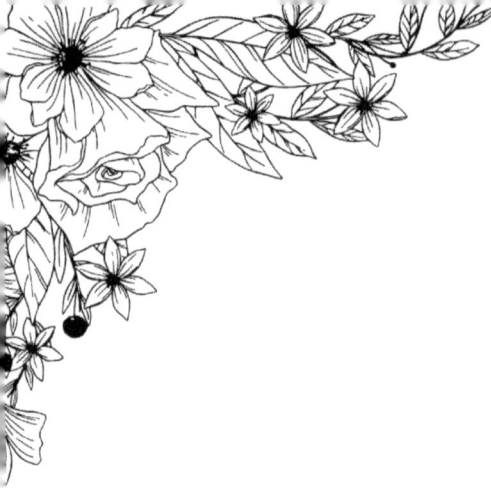

Do not rush through your healing!

(Healing is a journey, not a race)

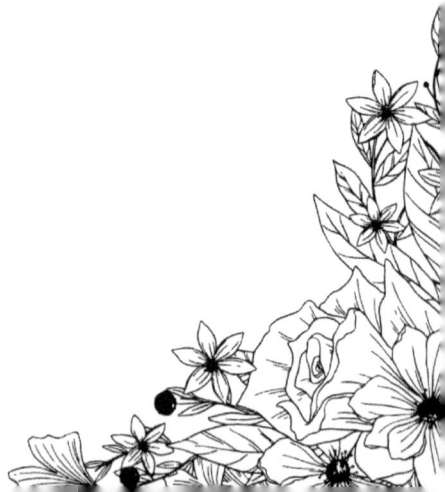

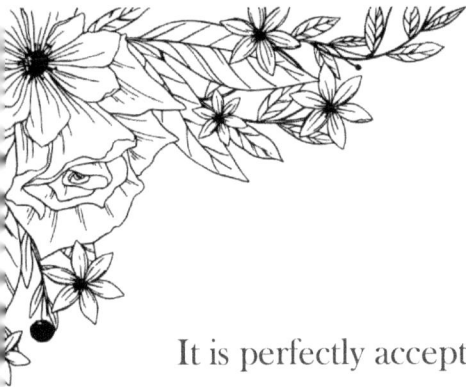

It is perfectly acceptable to ask for help!

Hey, you! Yes, you! Oh stubborn one, it is okay to ask for help!

Let me let you in on a little secret, we ALL need help! The trick is acknowledging this, understanding this, and accepting this!

Another secret, the world works better when we stop making people feel bad about needing help and being more compassionate because we never know when we will need it! It is okay to ask for help!

AND

It is okay to accept help!

If we could do everything on our own, then God would've given us all our own little islands, void of other people. We need each other more than we know!

Ask + Accept!

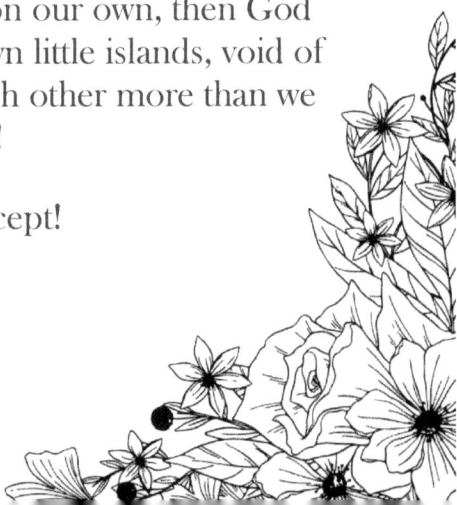

Do not look for your healing in the same place you lost your wholeness.

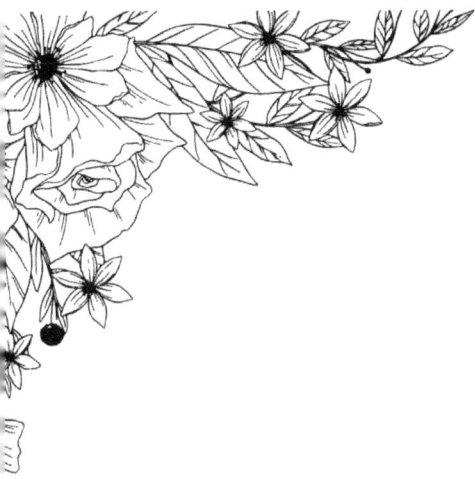

# Me Time:

Take it as often as you need to.

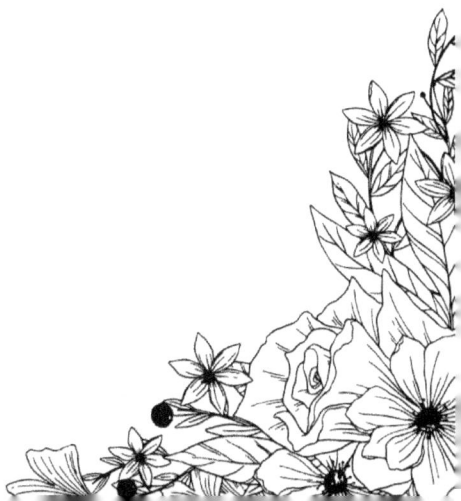

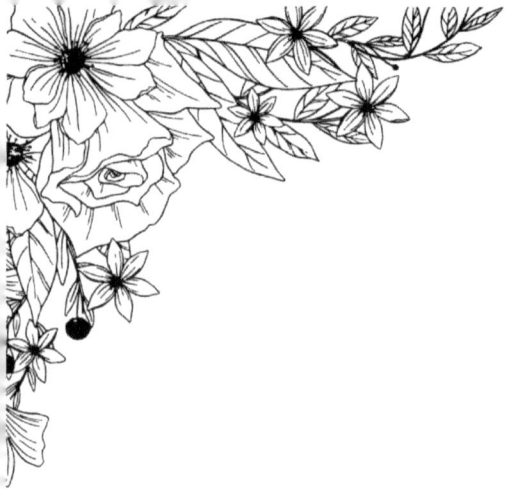

Be careful who you show your light to. Some people want to steal it from you!

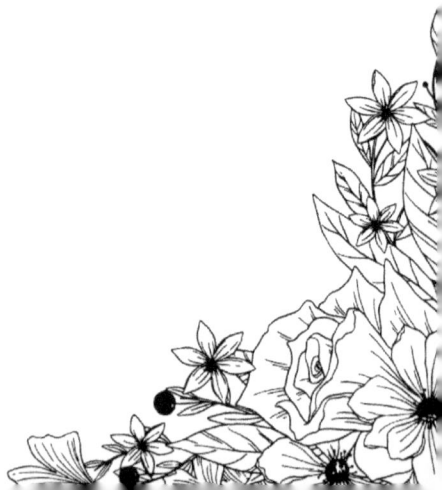

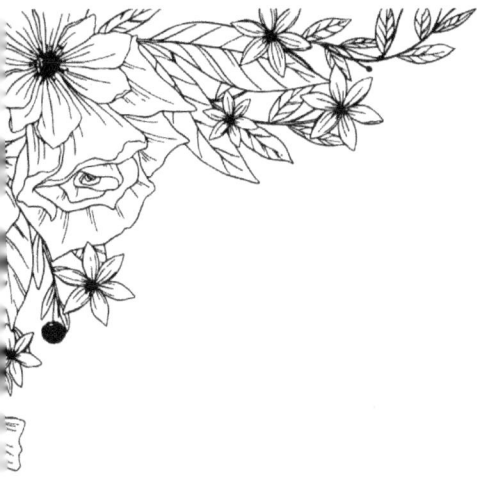

Set expectations for yourself!

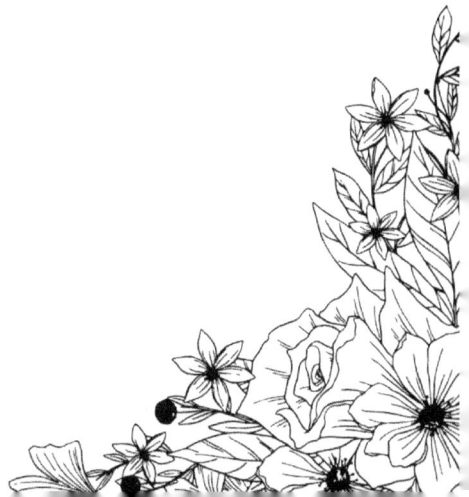

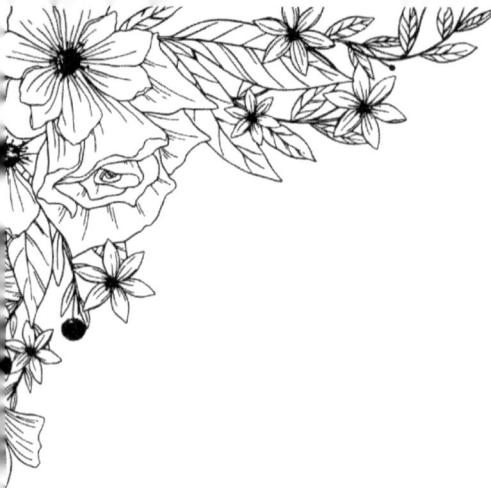

## QUALITY

————————

## QUANTITY

-My philosophy for life.

You do not need a lot to have a beautiful life.

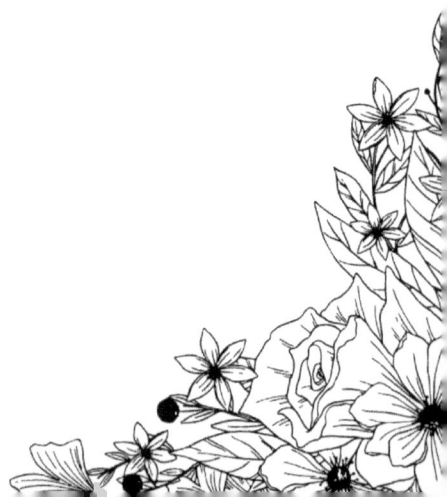

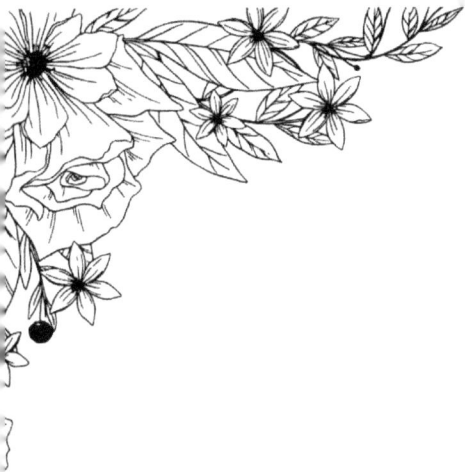

Enjoy the season you are currently experiencing.

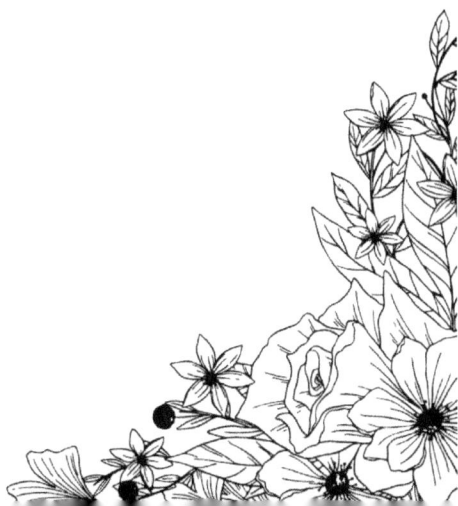

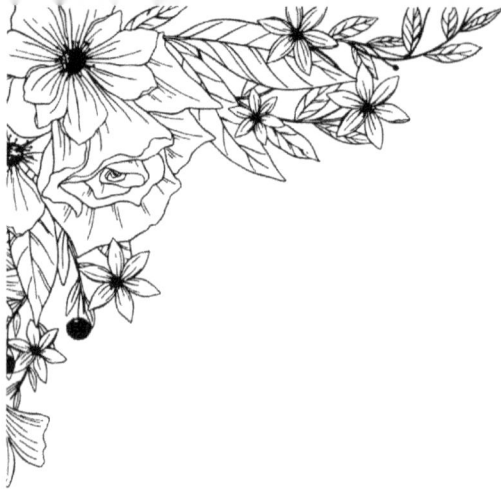

Deal.

Then heal.

So you can rebuild.

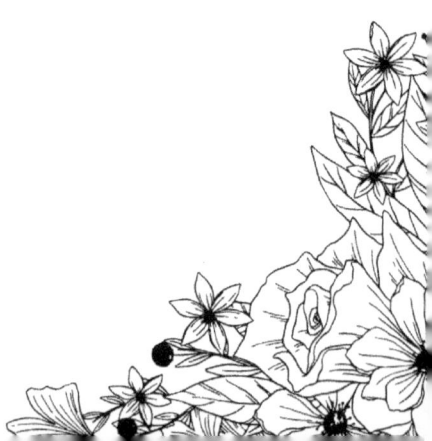

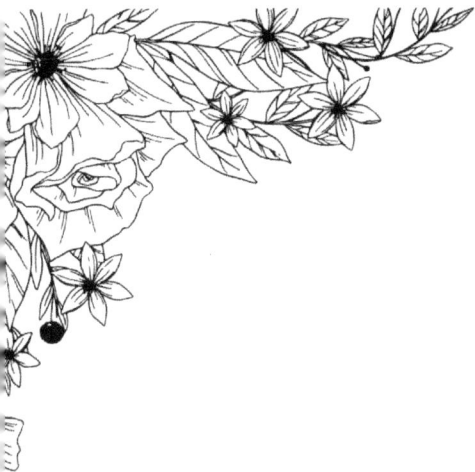

In a world where comparison is everything, I must tell myself, every day, that I am enough just the way I am.

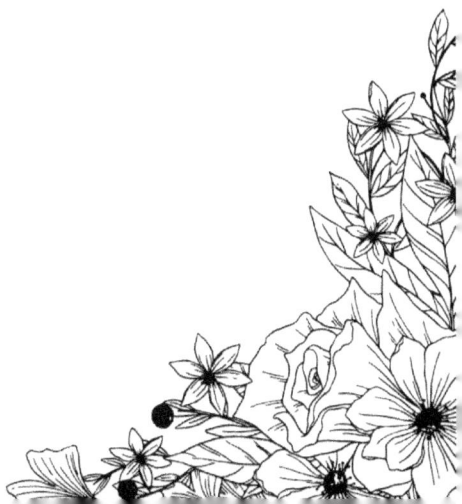

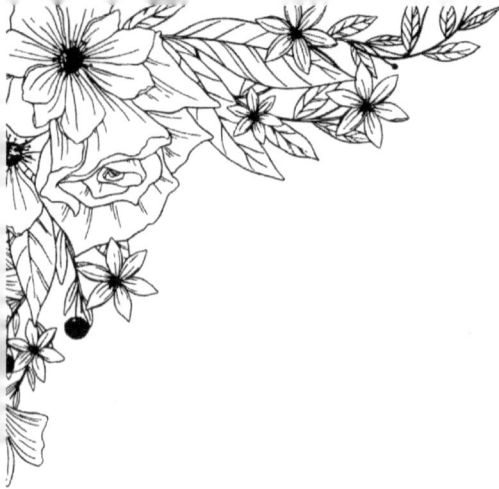

Stop criticizing yourself more than you praise yourself!

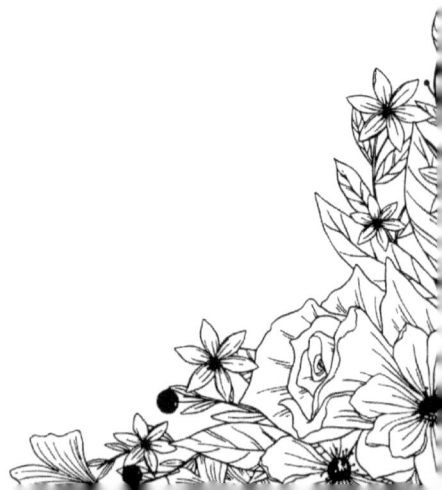

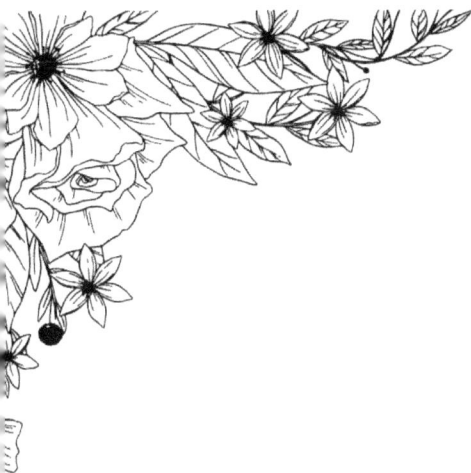

I no longer subscribe to being half loved.

I cancelled that subscription a long time ago.

Love me fully or leave me alone.

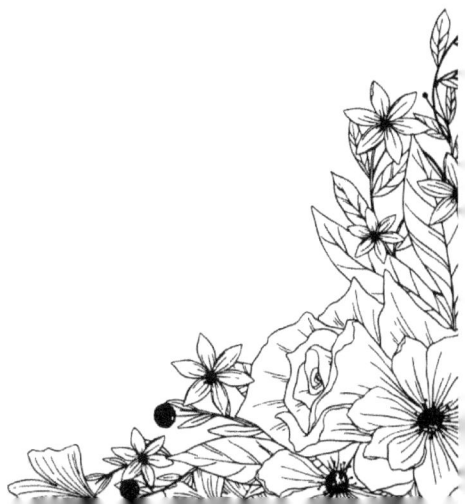

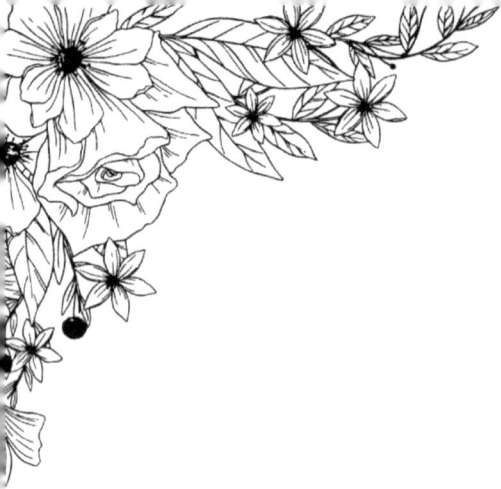

Please stop letting people mistreat you just because
they say they love you.

Love does not operate like that!

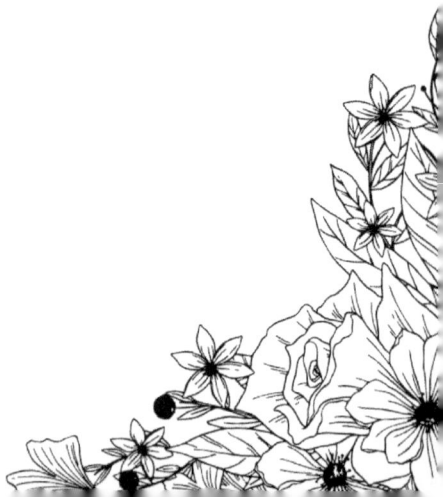

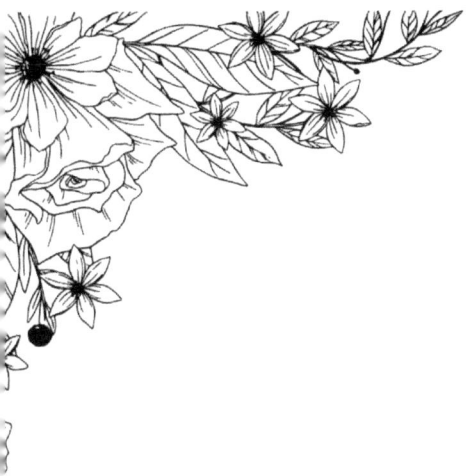

There is so much to wish for in this life, but there are even more things to be thankful for!

Have you identified your blessings today?

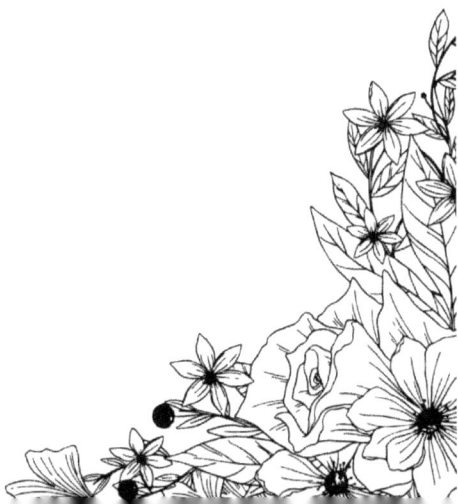

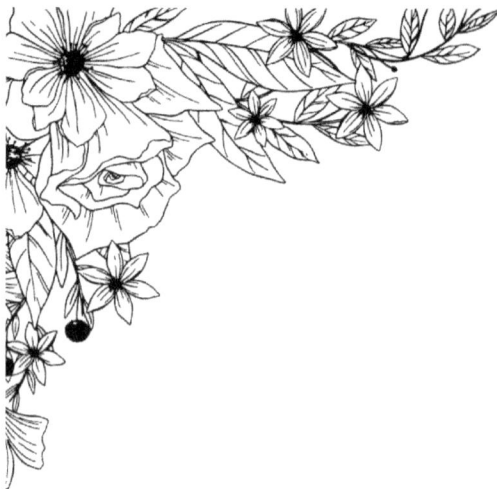

Dear Empaths + Highly Sensitive Persons,

Guard your heart and your soul.

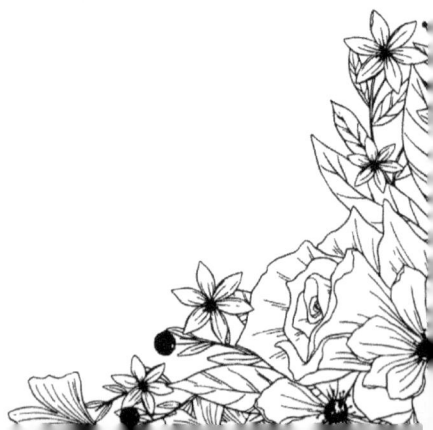

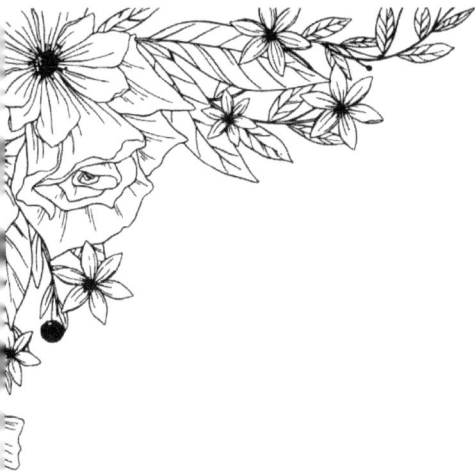

Focus on being YOUR best, not being THE best.

Competition kills creativity.

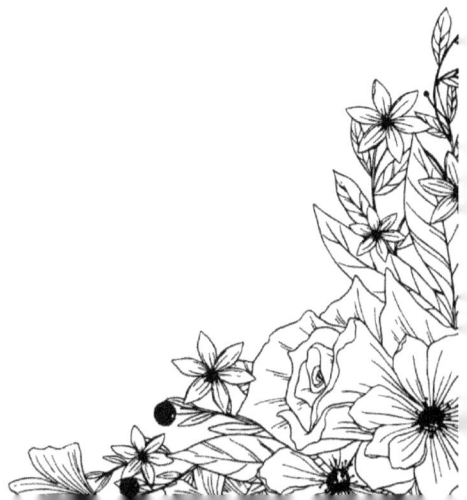

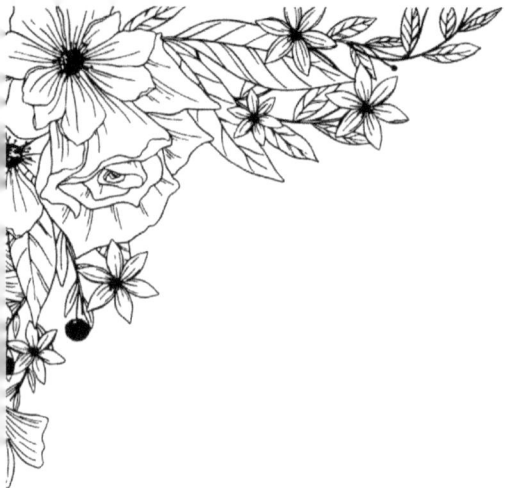

Make plans for your life, but do not plan your life.

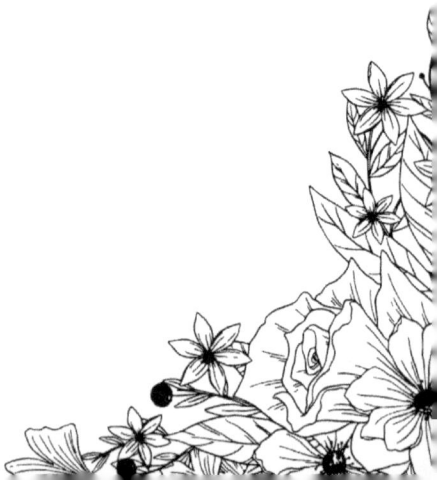

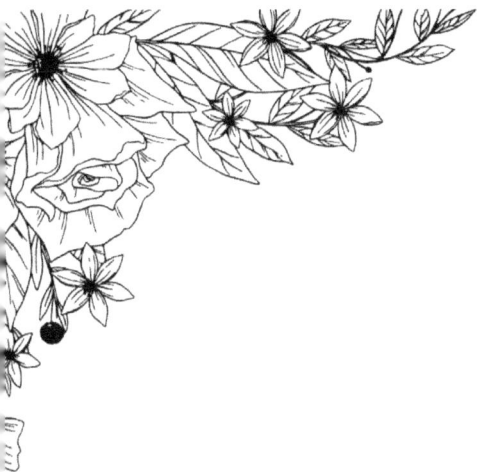

Do not be so worried about others that you forget
to check in on yourself.

How are YOU doing?

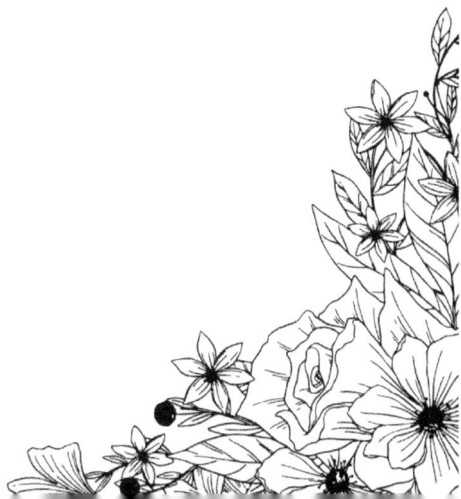

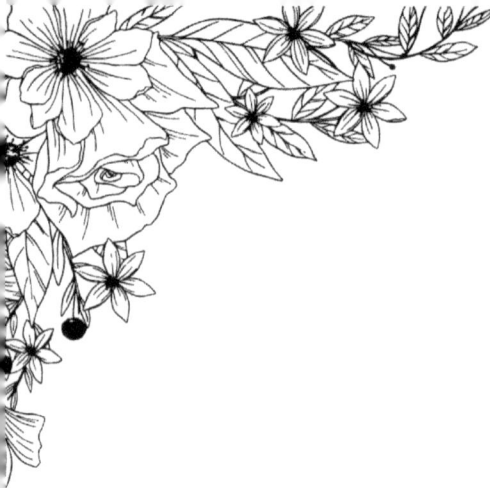

What is happening RIGHT NOW?

Check in with yourself at this moment.

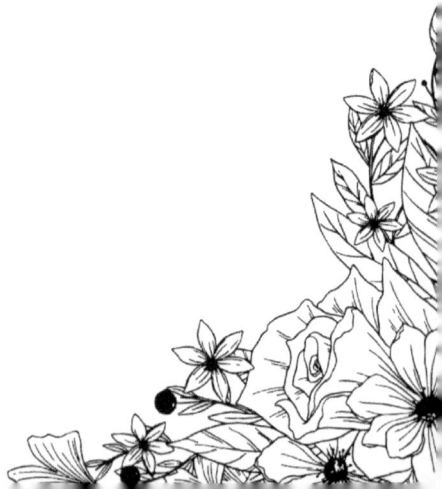

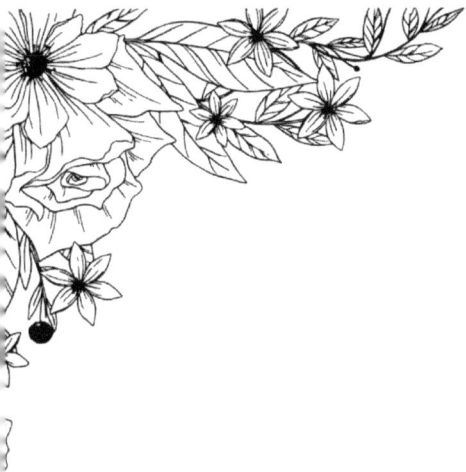

Just Breathe

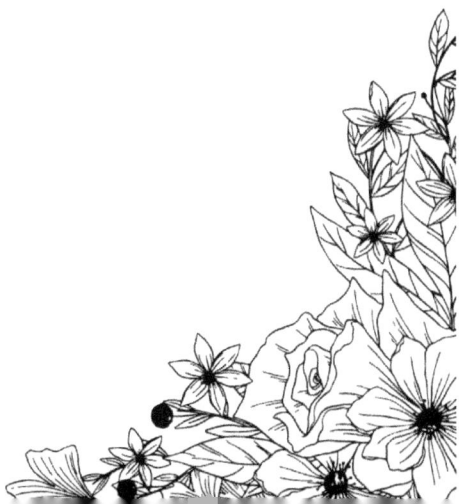

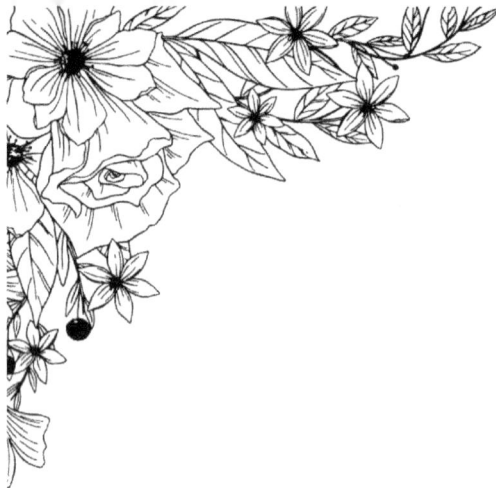

When was the last time you dug to the bottom of your purse (soul)?

-While cleaning out my purse, one day, I found everything I needed at the bottom. I wonder what I would find if I dug deep into my soul.

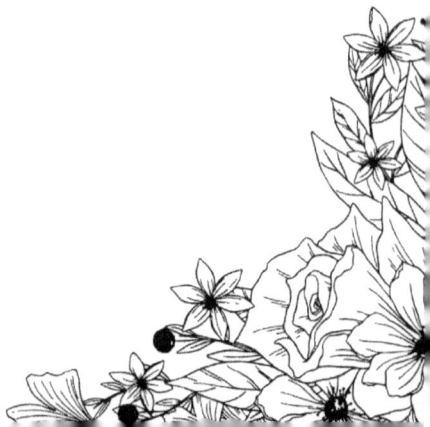

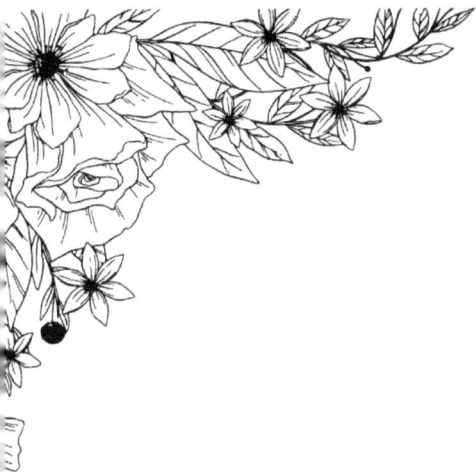

May your soul find peace and reside there forever.

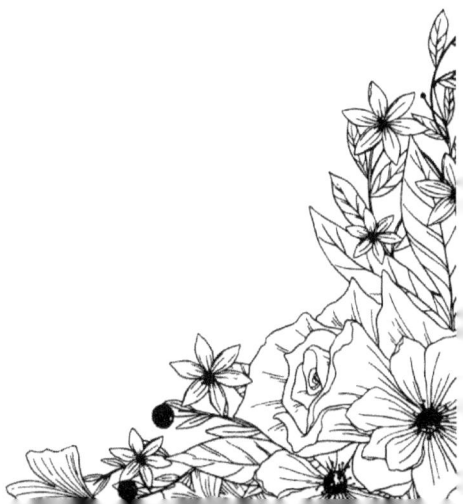

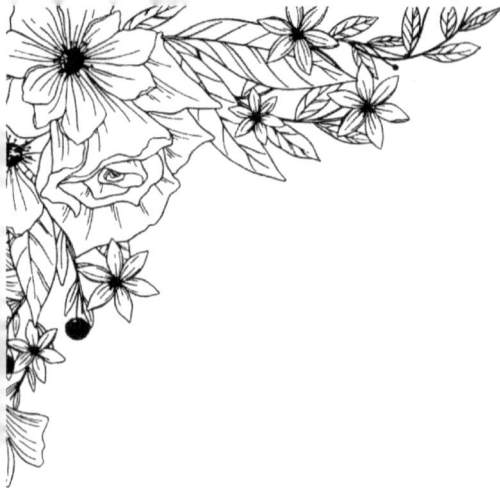

Stop planting your seeds of love in soil that will not help it grow!

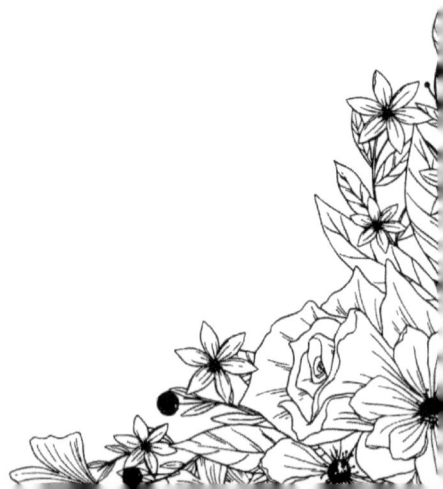

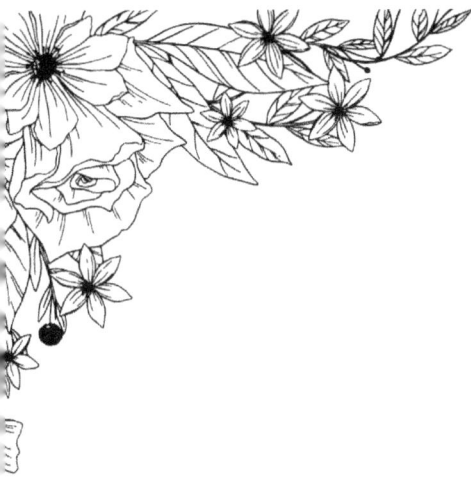

No.

(Believe it or not, that is a full sentence)

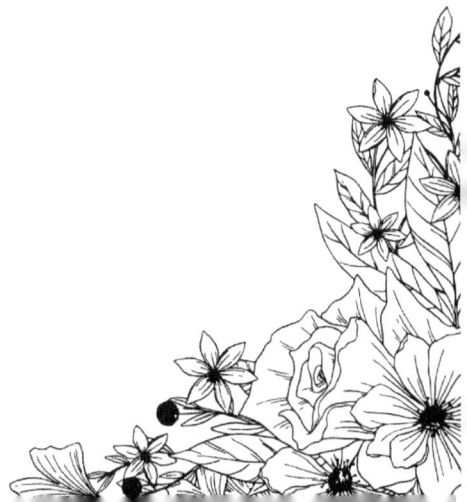

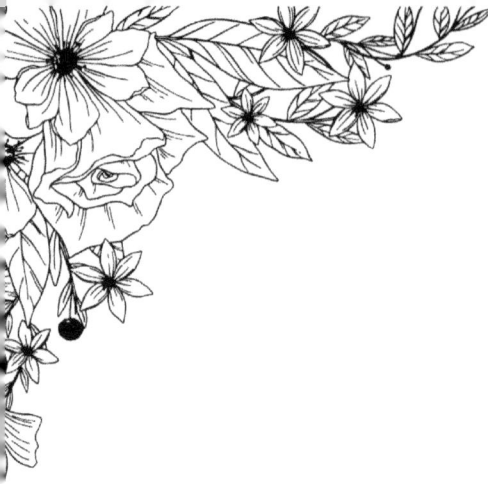

When was the last time your cup overflowed?

Always fill your own cup.

You cannot wait on others to do that for you.

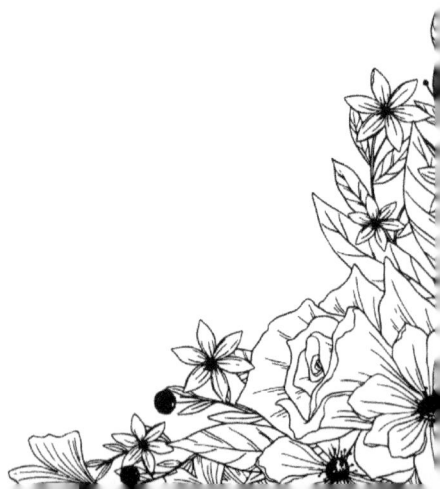

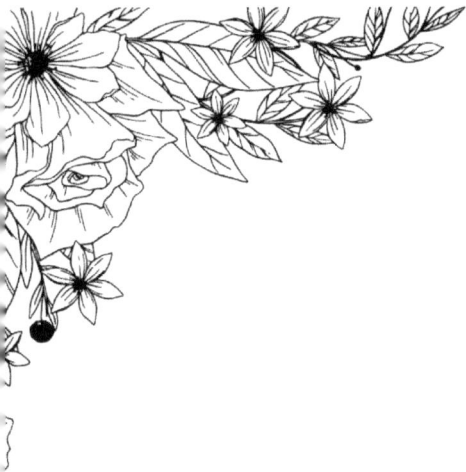

Today, I encourage you to dig deep for sunshine!

It is there.

Some days you just have to search a little bit harder.

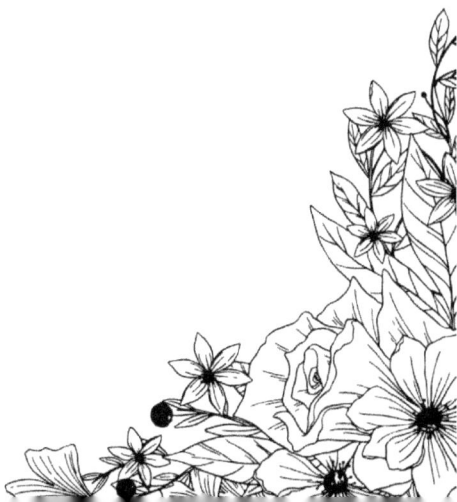

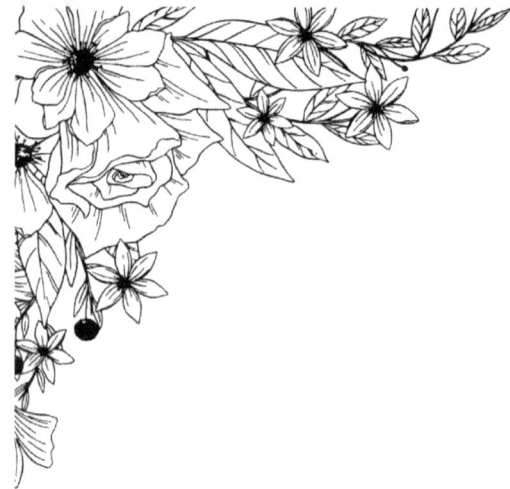

Gratitude.

(we all want what we do not have, until we get it,
then we want something else)

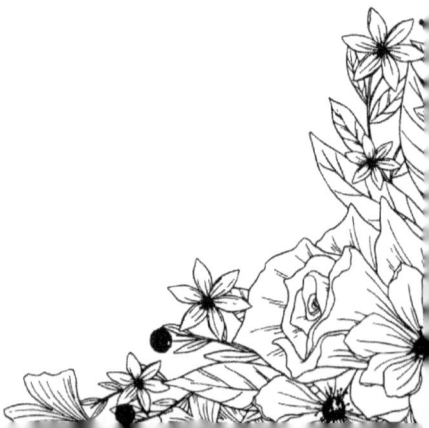

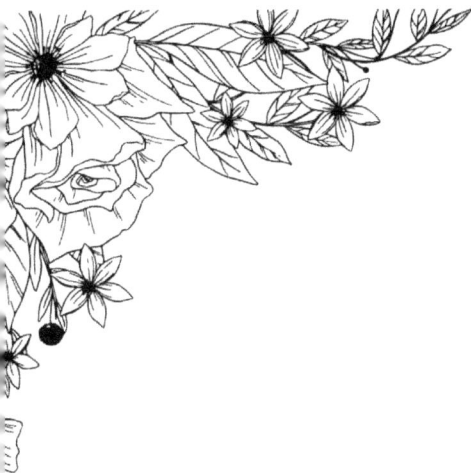

Your goal for every day:


Give Yourself Grace

+

Believe In Yourself

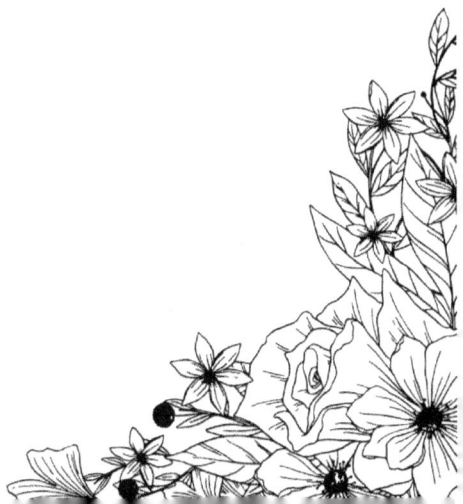

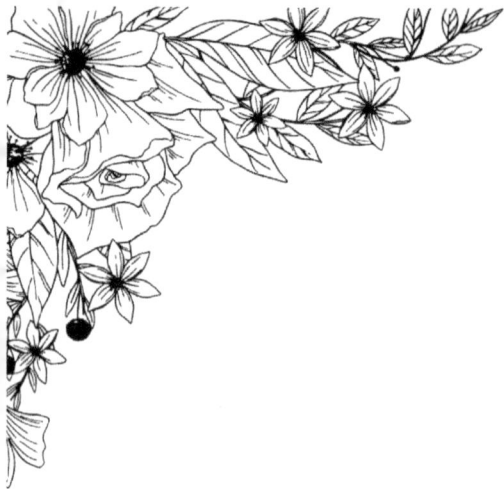

Not everyone deserves access to your energy.

Preserve it!

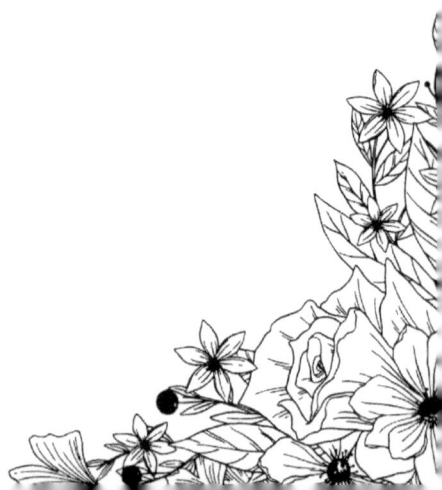

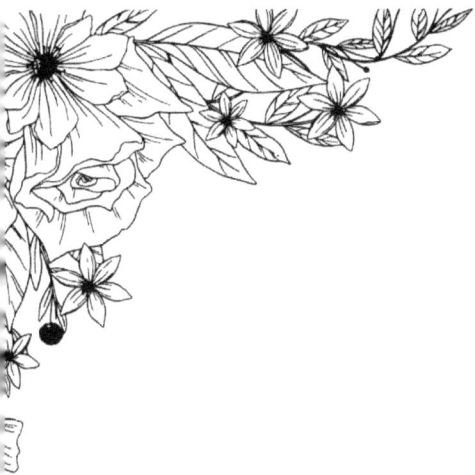

Being single does not mean you are broken.

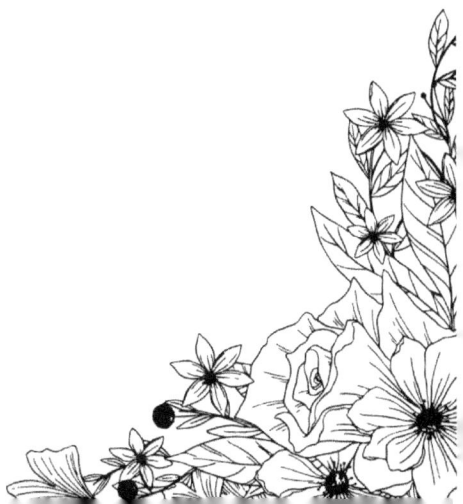

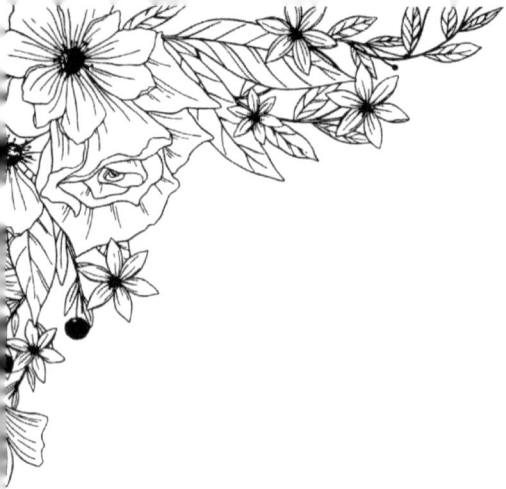

Affirm Yourself:

I am creating the life I deserve to live.

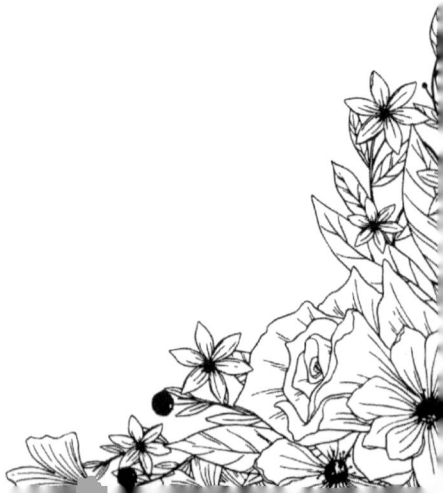

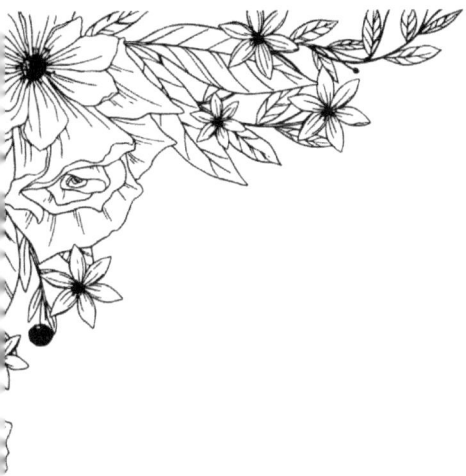

Heal + Grow

MY LOVE,

THIS IS YOUR MAIN PRIORITY.

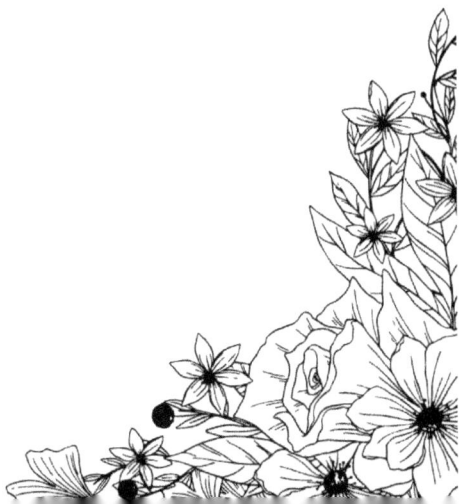

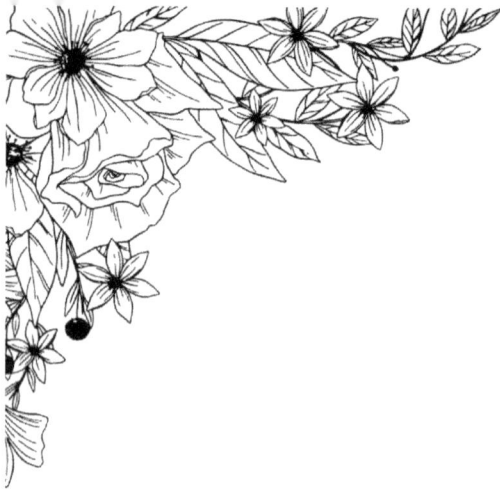

Happiness is not in the next best thing that happens to you; happiness is within.

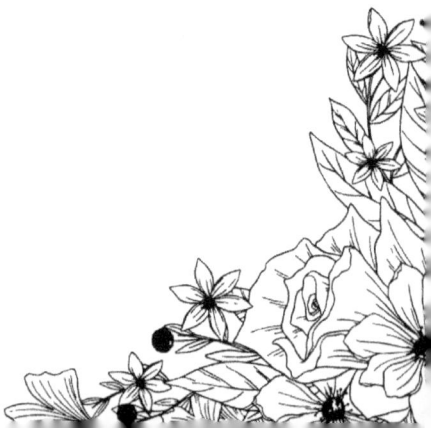

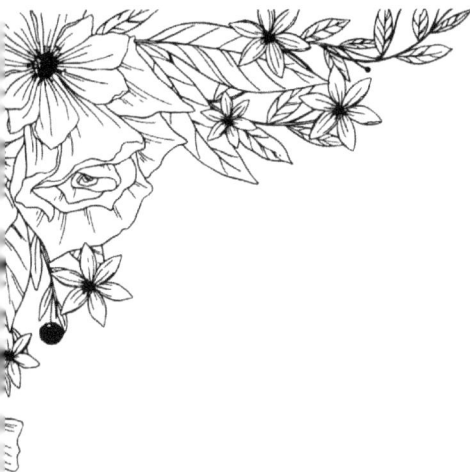

When you sign up to love someone, you must love the good and the bad. That is the job! You cannot choose which parts to love.

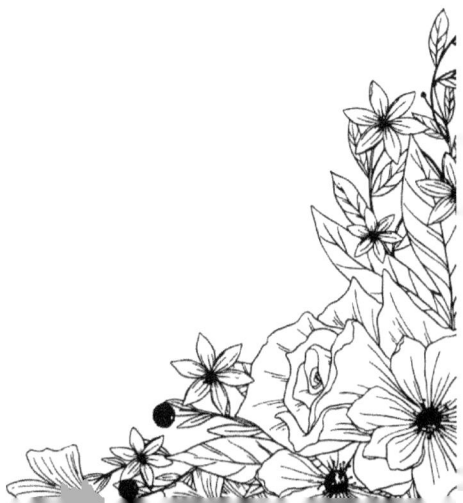

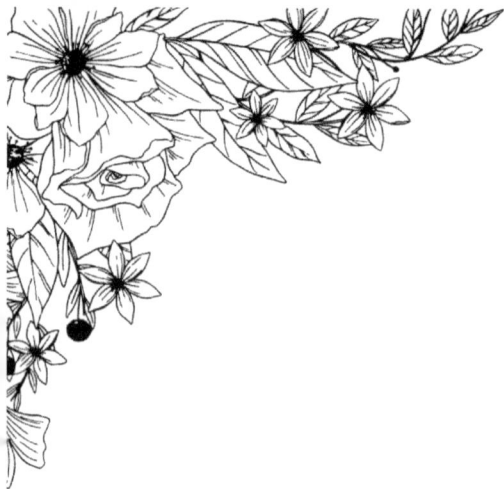

May we all learn to have peace within, so we can spread it without, freely and unconditionally.

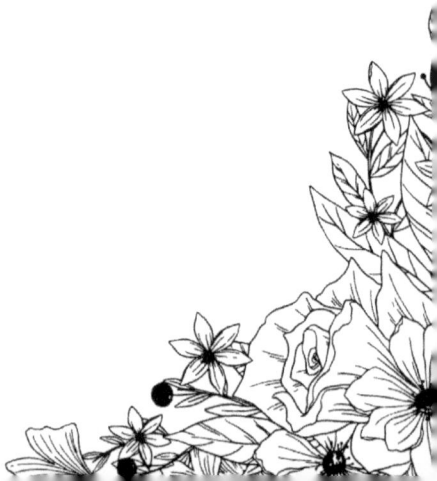

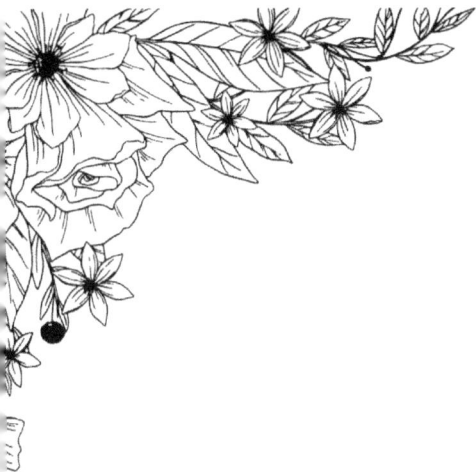

Mantra:

There is never a day that I wake up, where I am not
the prize. I am always the prize.

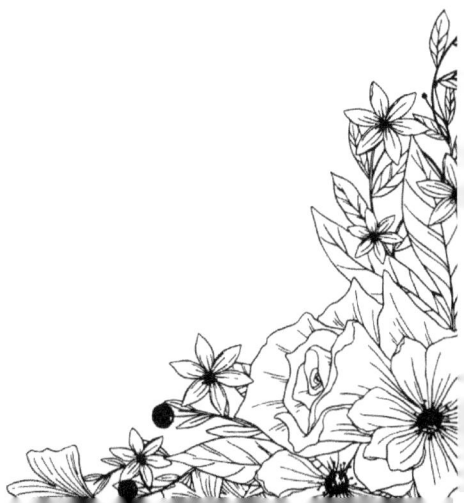

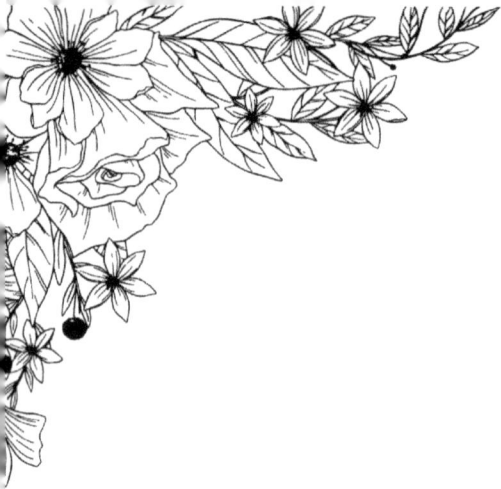

Next time, I am keeping some of me!

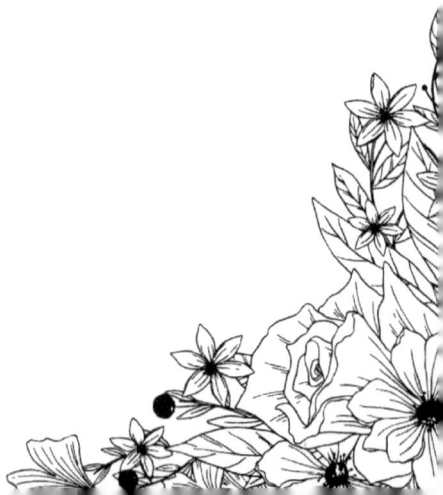

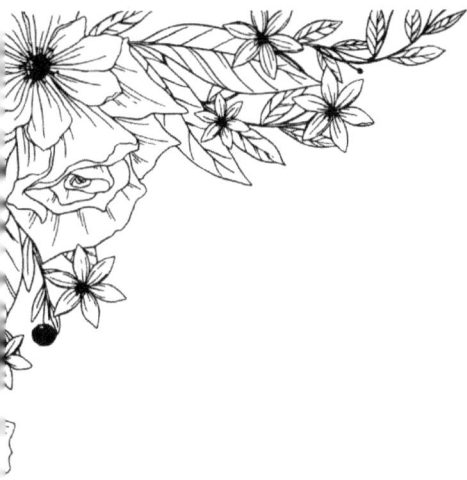

My current situation IS NOT my permanent situation.

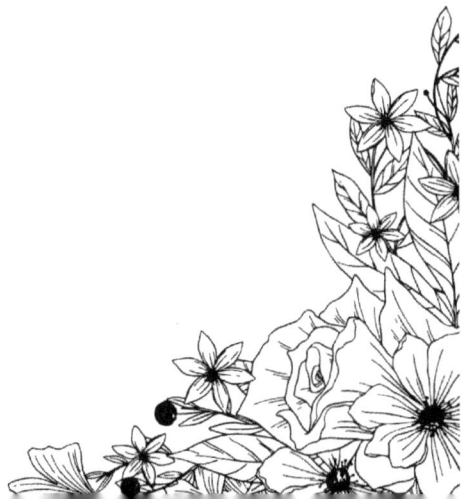

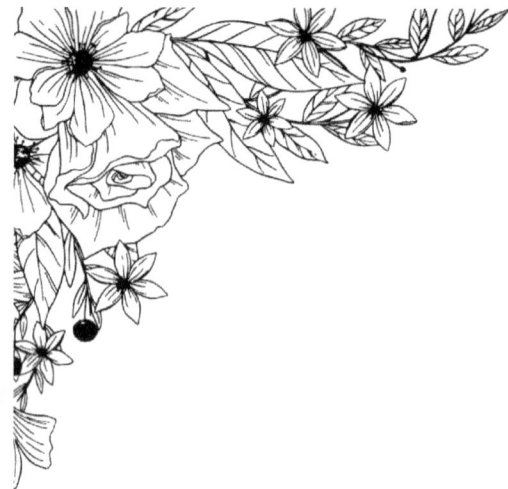

Activity:

Write a letter to your ex/exes.

*Hear me out, you do not have to give it to them. Just purge, burn it, and release.*

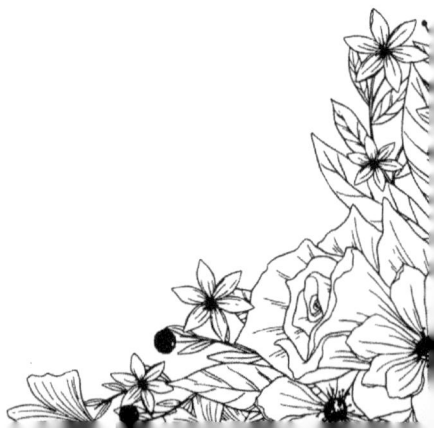

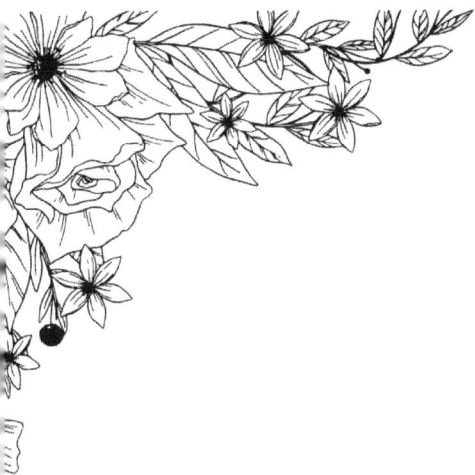

I do not get to choose how someone else chooses to love me, but I do get to choose whether I will accept it or not.

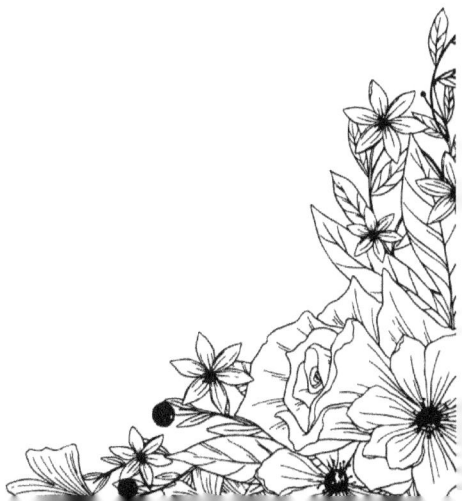

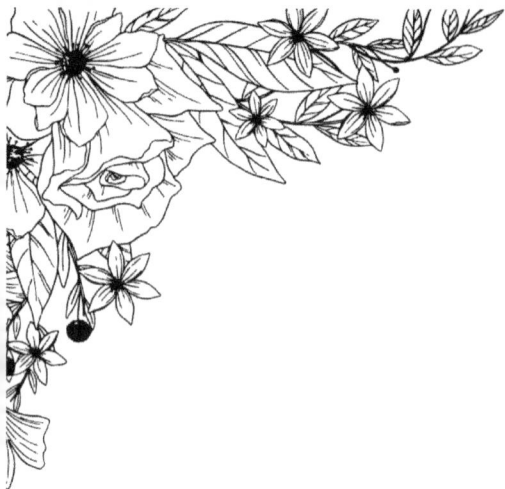

Breathe. So you can achieve.

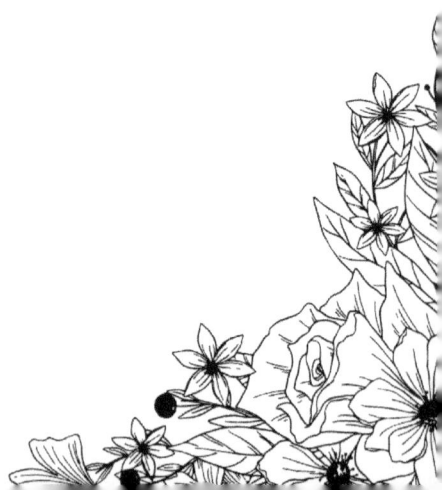

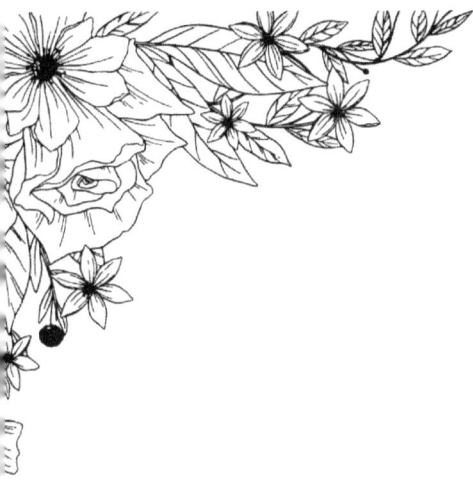

Please stop trying to be everything to everyone.

It is not possible, and it is exhausting!

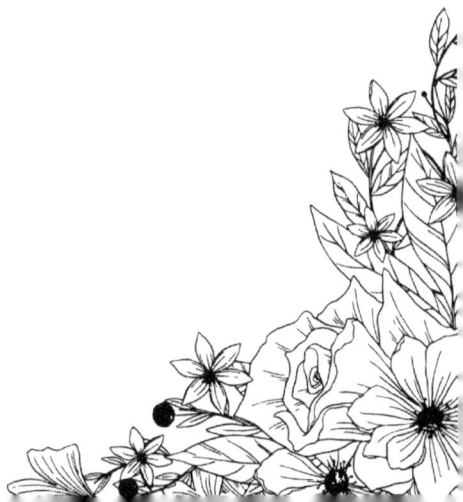

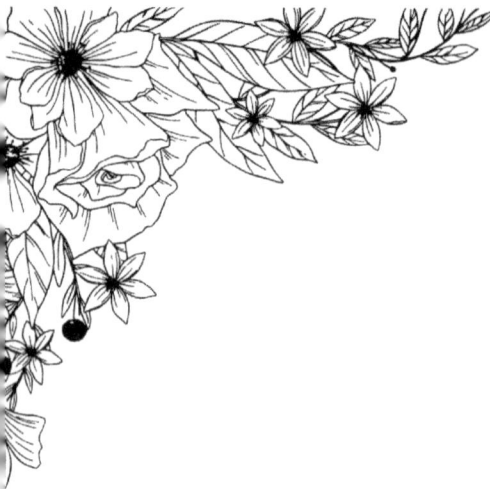

Focus on the present because the future is not yet
ready for us!

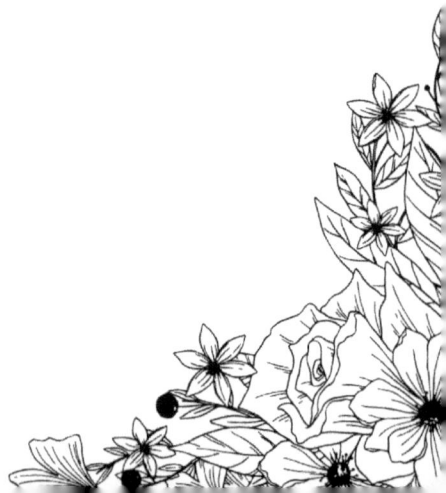

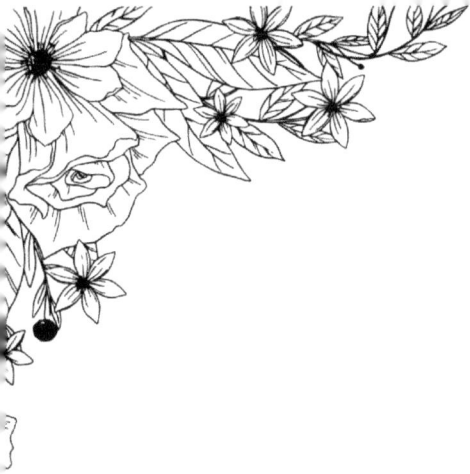

It is easier to be hesitant than hopeful, but I am begging you to choose hope!

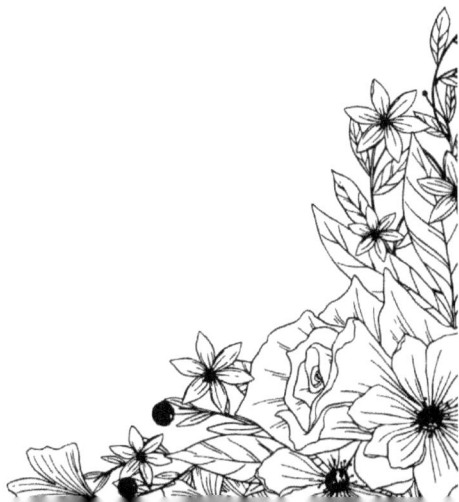

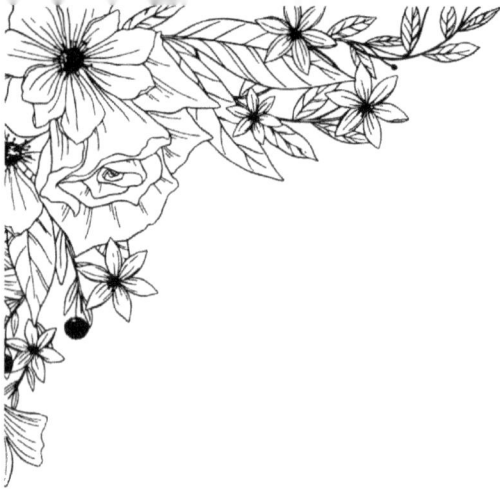

Please stop telling people you are there for them,
when who you need to be there for is yourself.

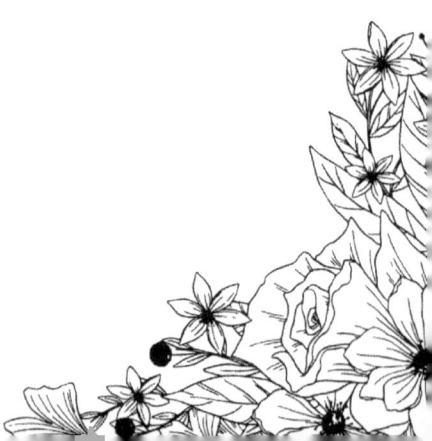

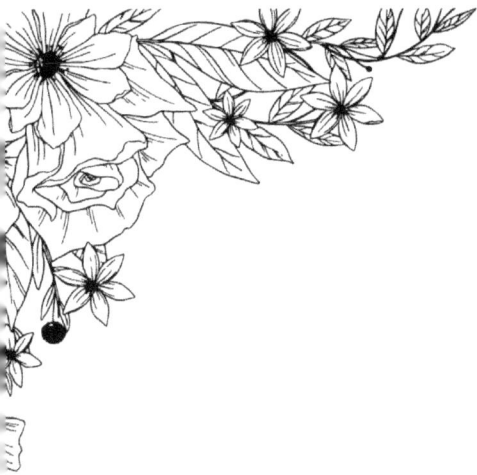

People come and go, but my love for myself is forever.

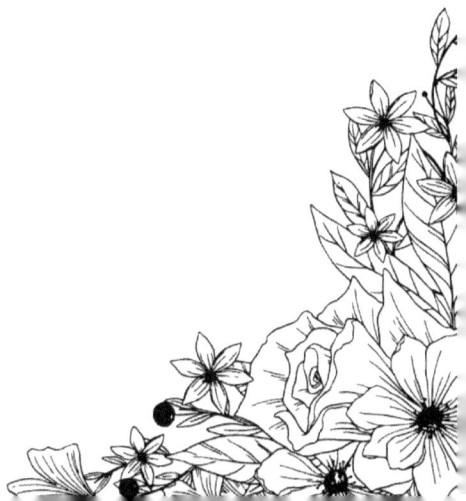

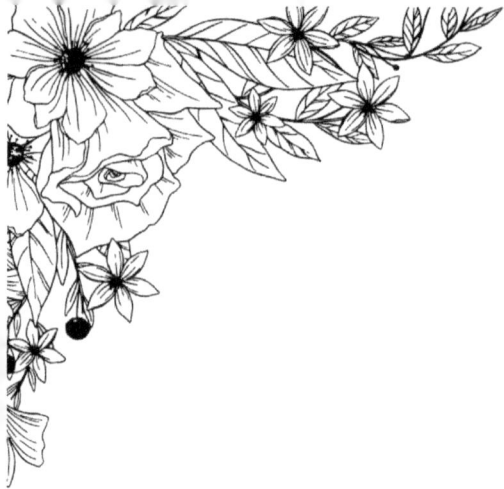

It is better to be alone than guess how someone feels about you!

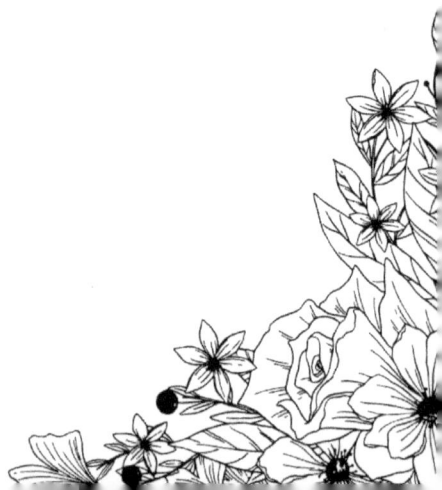

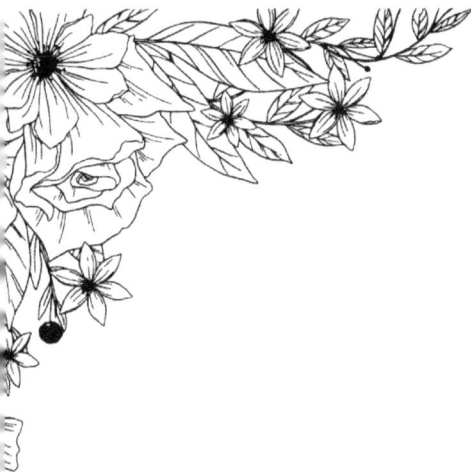

Never apologize for your purpose.

Walk fully in it.

It is yours for a reason.

Not everyone will understand it

And that is okay.

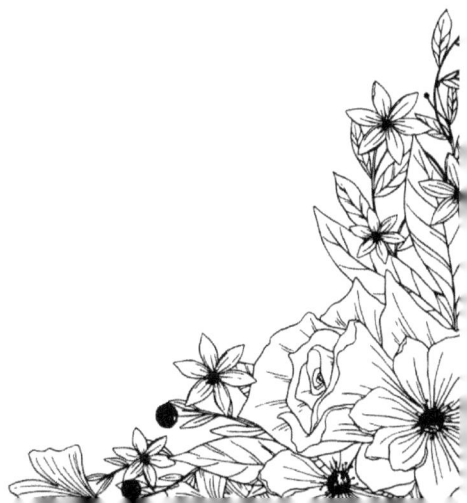

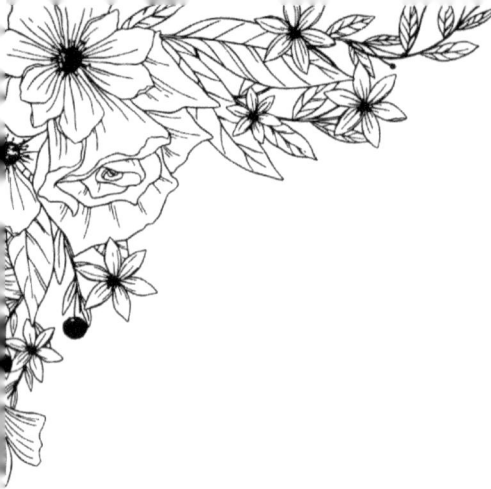

Stop wishing your life away.

Be present in the moment.

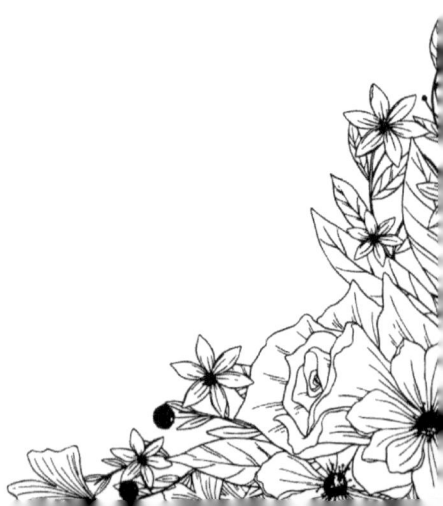

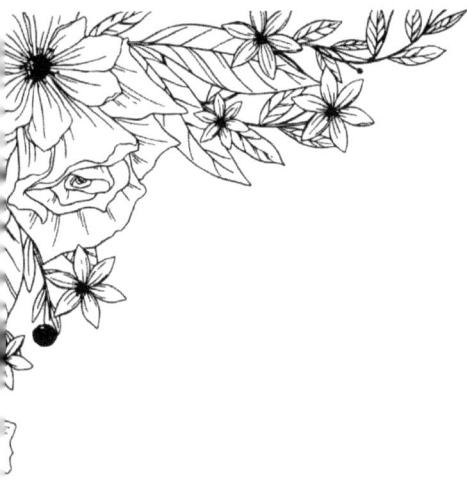

Do not allow someone to make you feel bad for
loving + appreciating yourself.

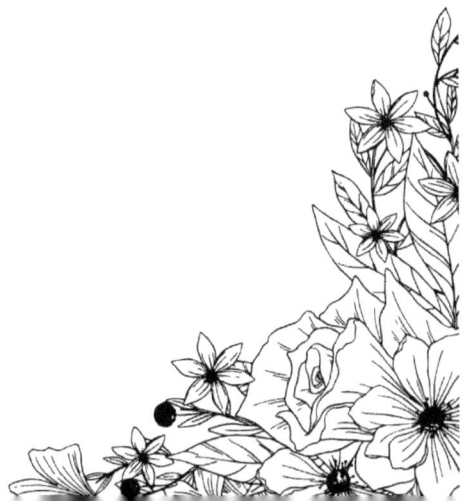

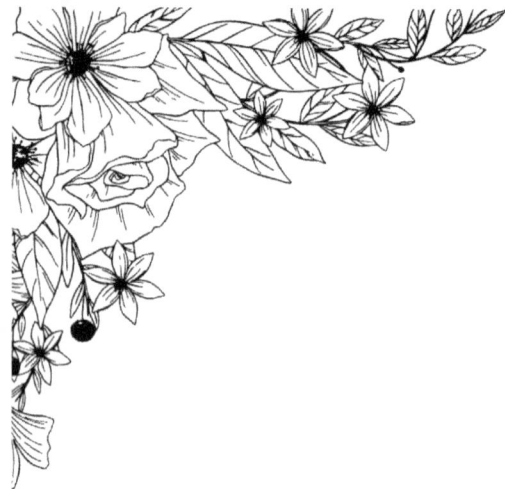

Who taught you to think so little of yourself?

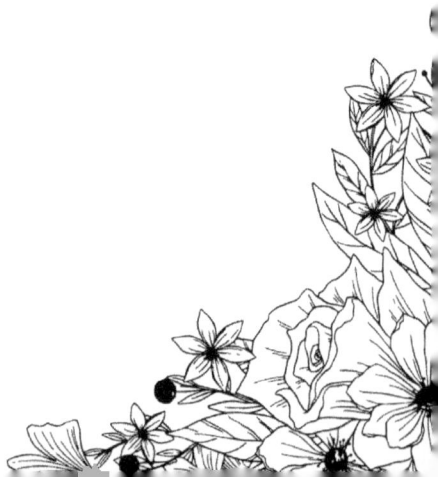

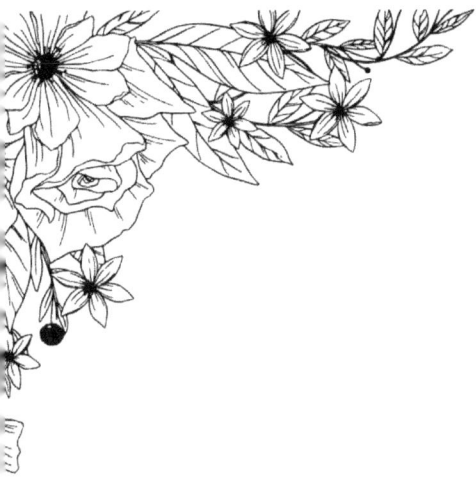

Why are worried about later?

Later does not care about us.

Focus on now.

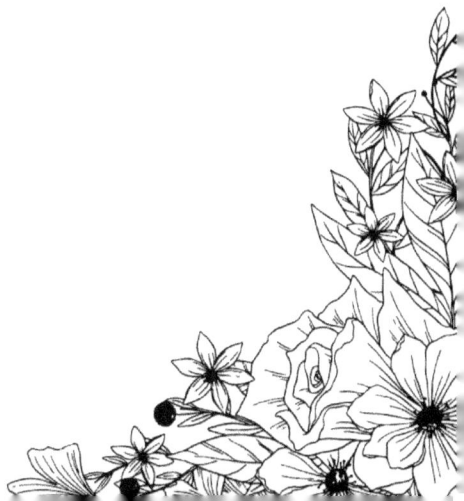

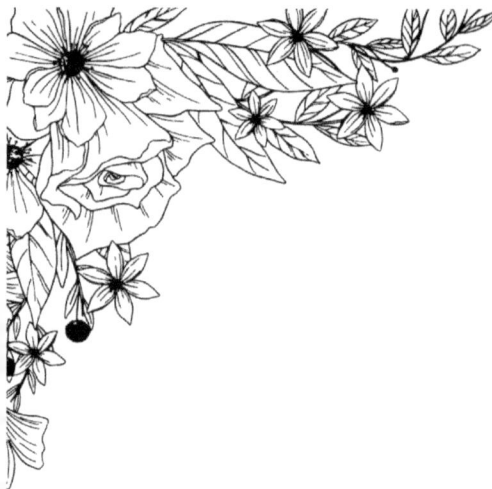

Do not worry about love finding you.

Be more concerned with losing the love you have for yourself.

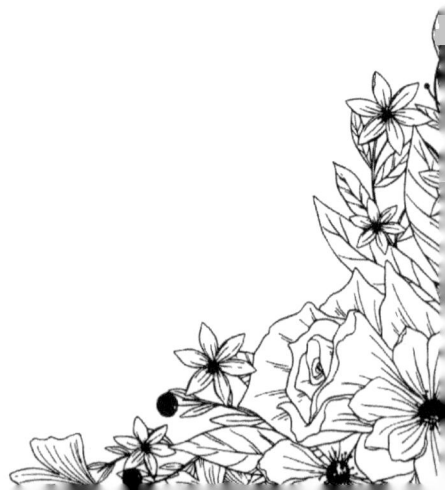

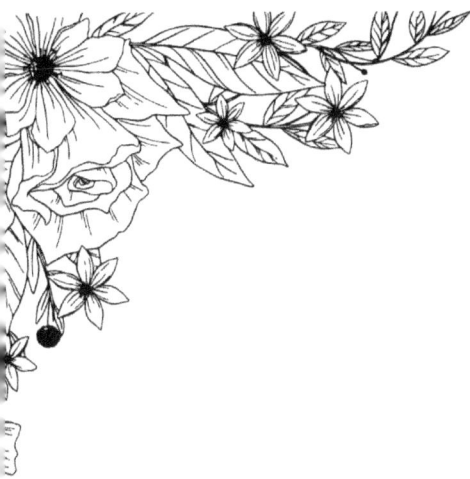

Do not continue allowing people to withdraw from your emotional bank, without depositing something.

You deserve to be emotionally full.

Stop letting people emotionally bankrupt you.

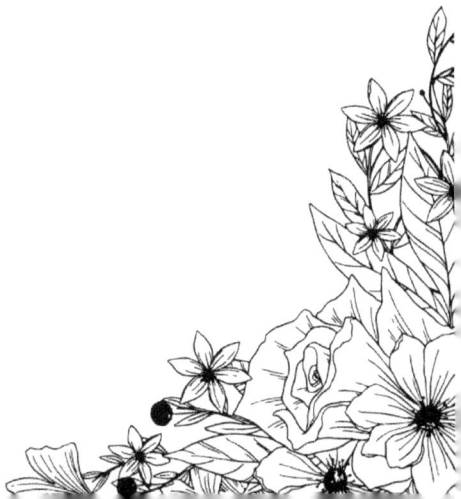

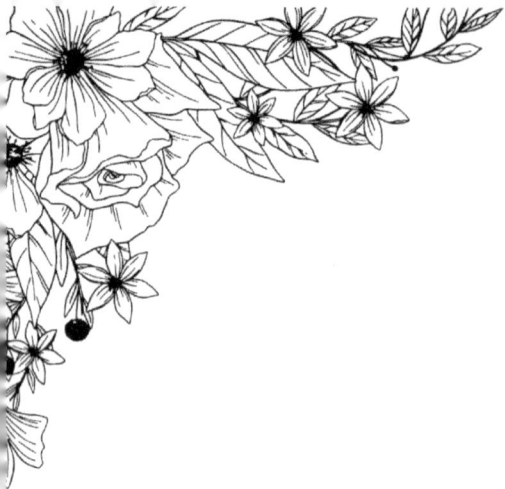

Stop doubting yourself!

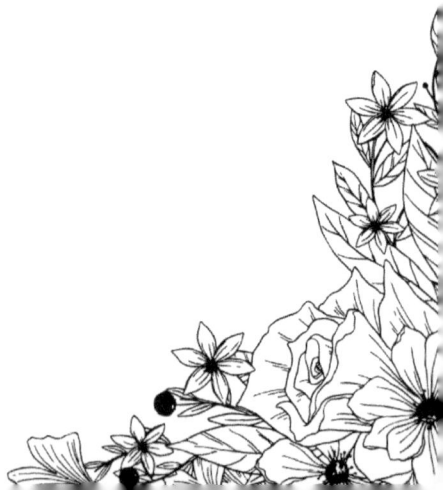

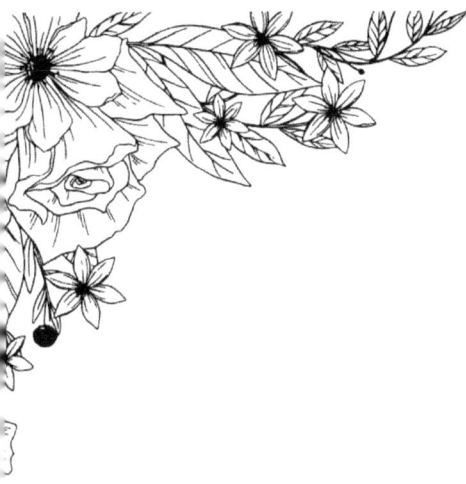

Two emotions can exist within you at the same time!

No one is a solitary feeler.

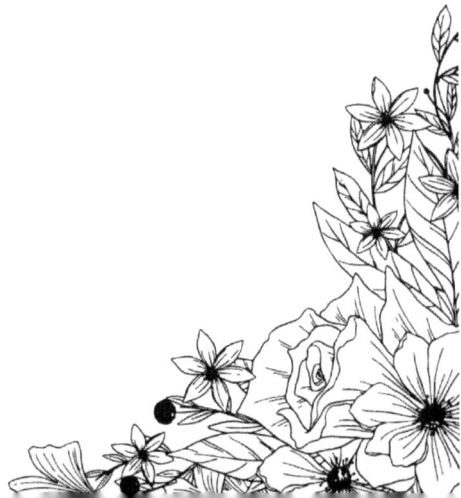

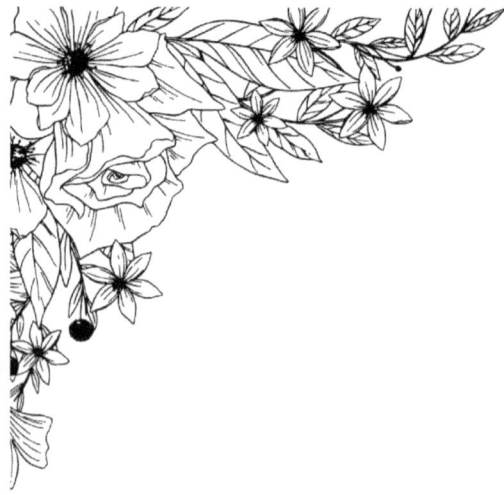

You must first see the good in yourself before you can see it in others!

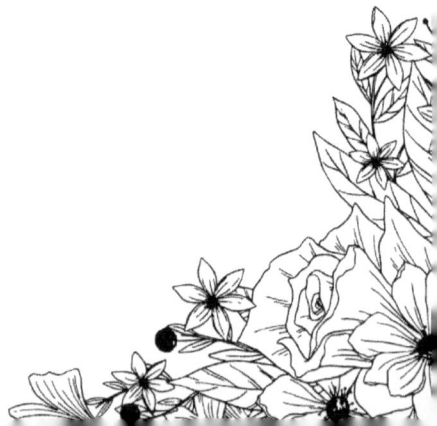

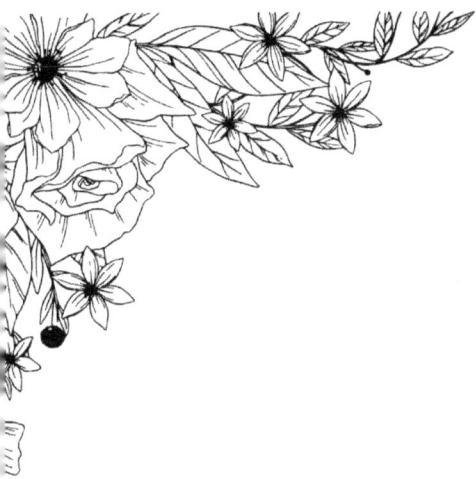

It is impossible to hate others when you love yourself!

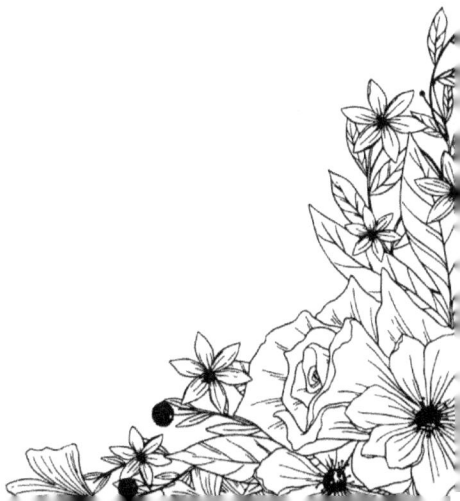

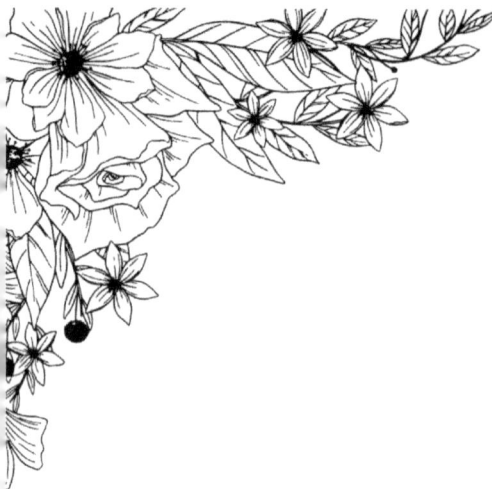

Stop using your past as a point of reference for your future!

Spoiler Alert: You are not going back there!

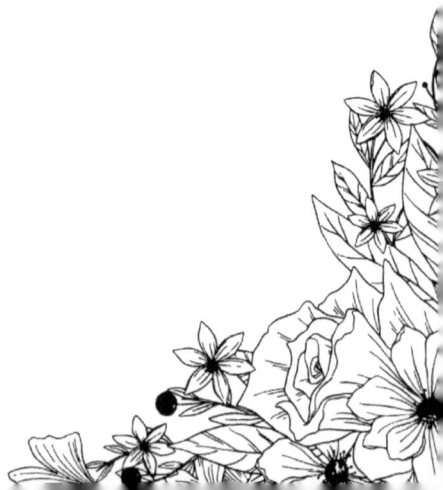

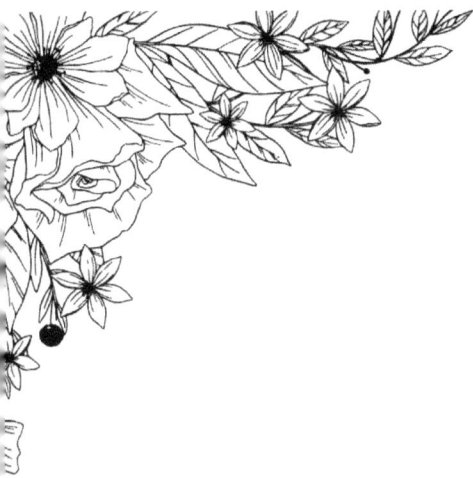

When you love yourself, people's perceptions of you become unimportant. When you love your flaws and all, there is very little a person can make you feel bad about who you are.

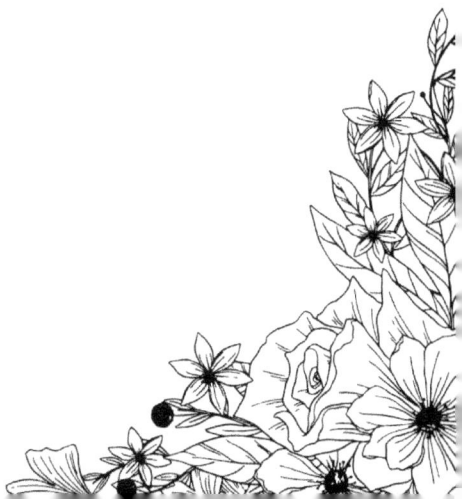

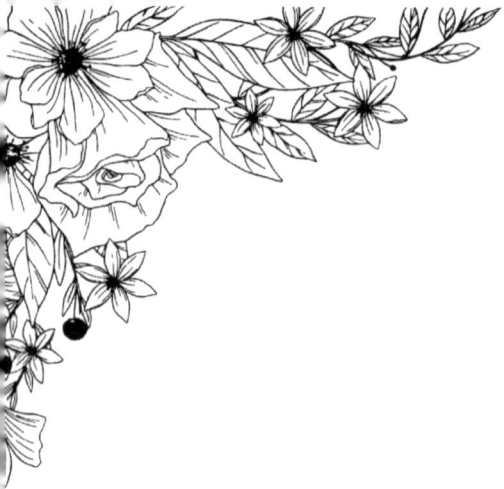

If a person is not adding to you, then they are taking from you. I encourage you to take inventory of your life. See where your energy is going and then see if it is being returned to you!

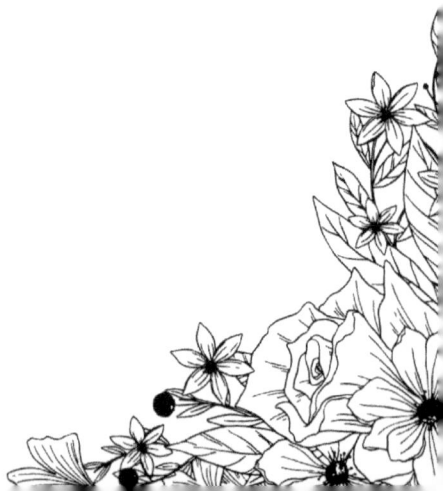

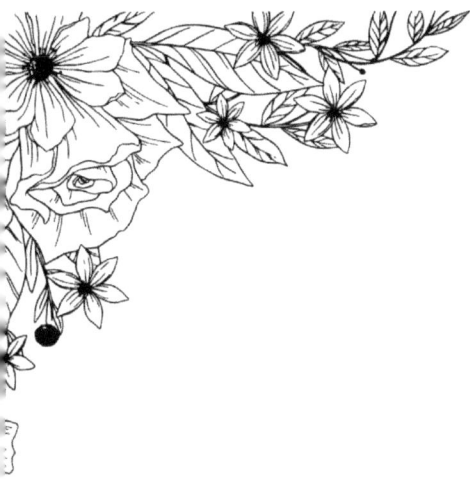

Are you not tired of punishing yourself?

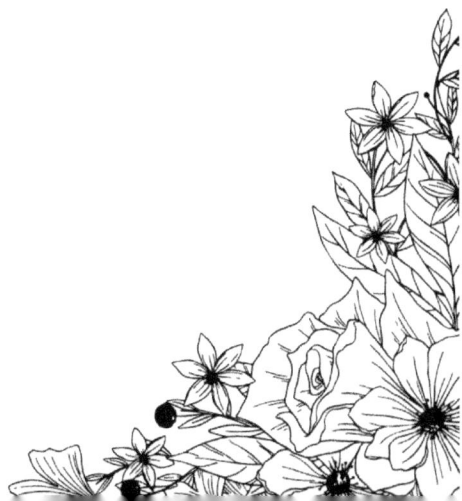

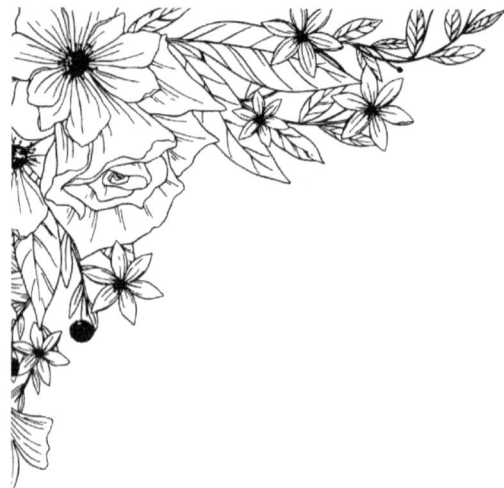

When you have the need to seek attention and acceptance from EVERYONE, you will NEVER be comfortable with yourself!

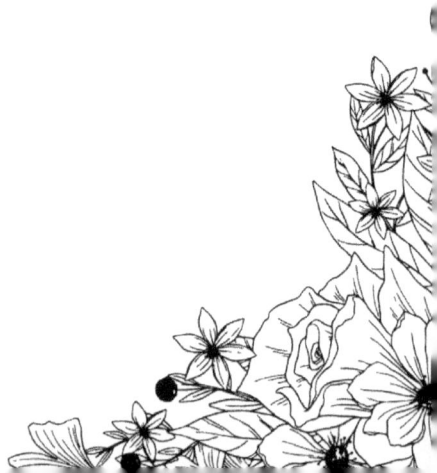

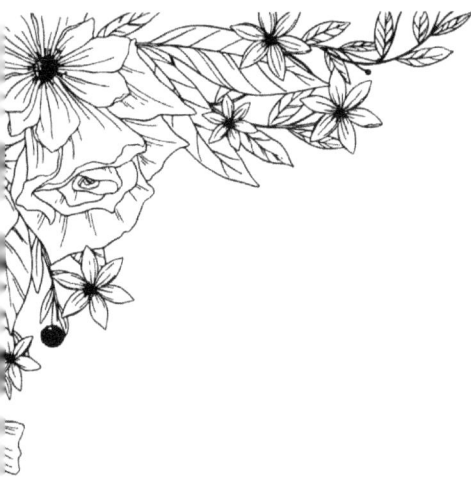

Sometimes fear causes you to see things that are not there. Stop sabotaging yourself!

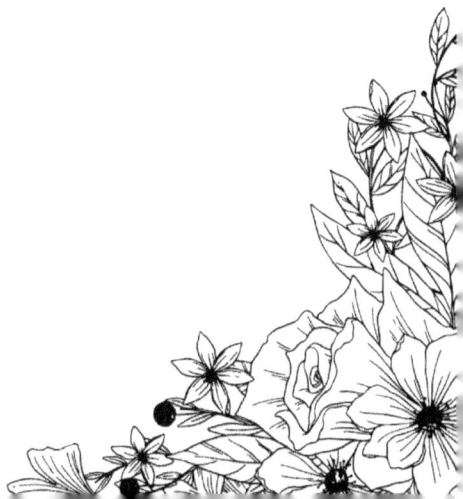

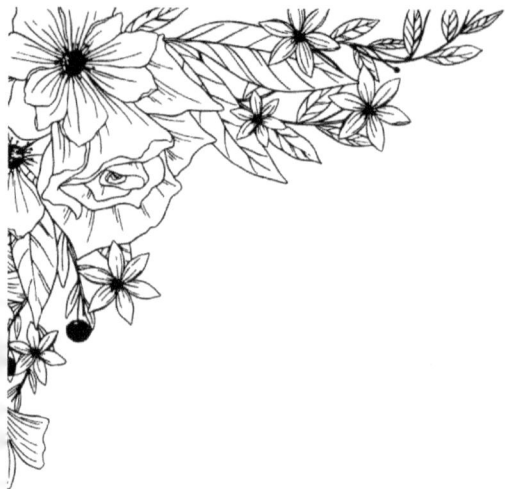

Stop allowing yesterday's mistakes and tomorrow's
worries take away today's joy!

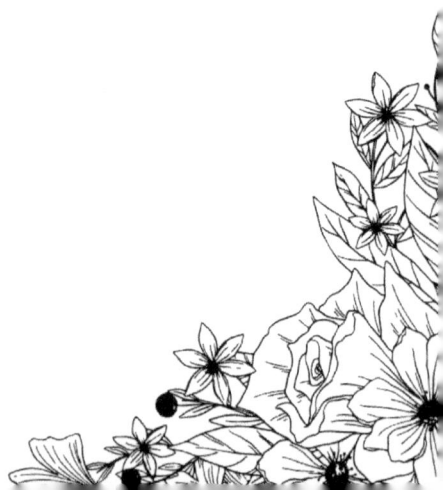

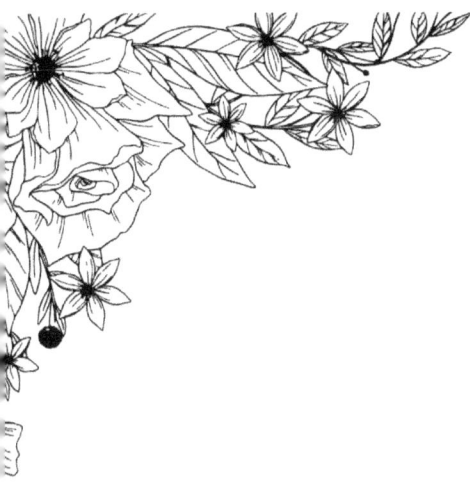

An incomplete person will never possess the necessary tools to complete someone else.

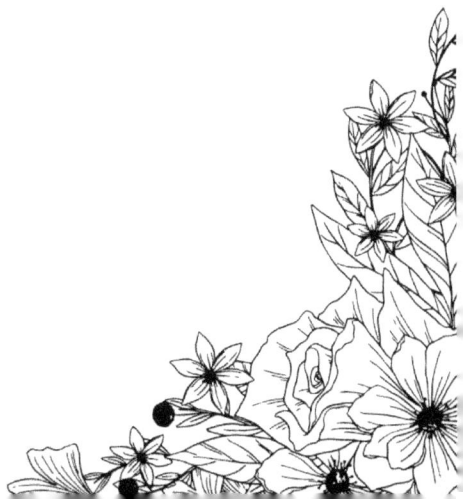

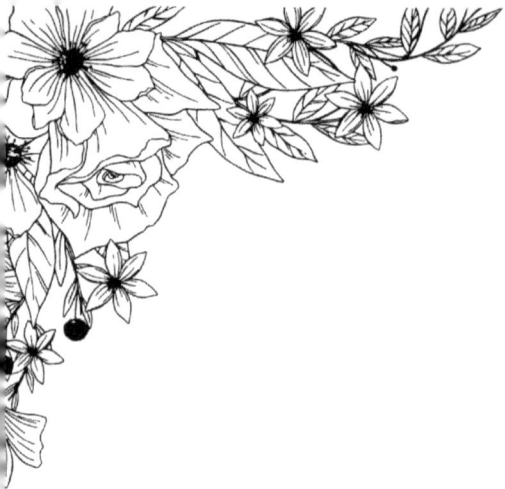

No one can make me feel ashamed of who I USE to be. I love the old me because she destroyed me and made me who I am today. I could never thank her enough.

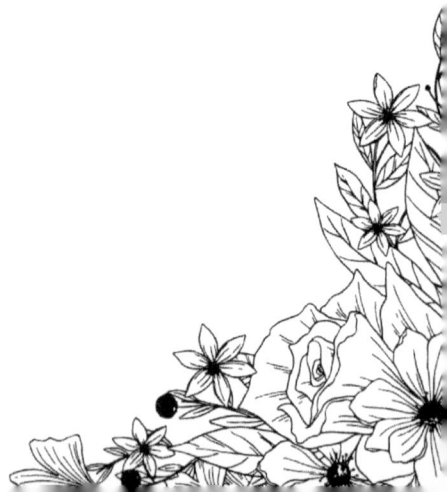

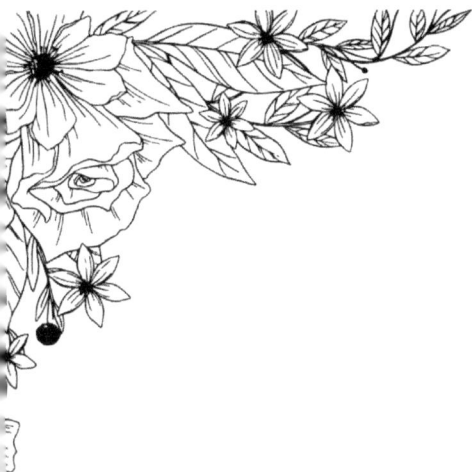

I have spent the majority of my life being unhappy, so you will have to excuse me if I do not want to participate in activities that do not foster peace of mind.

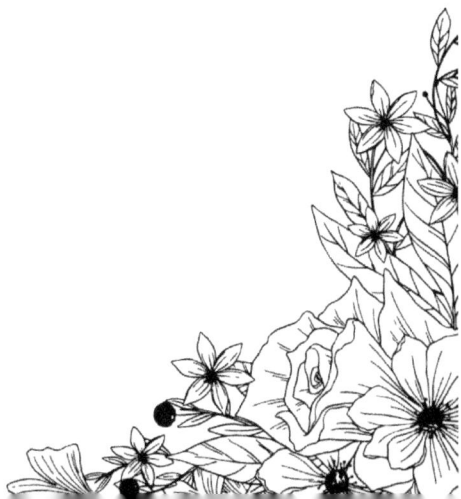

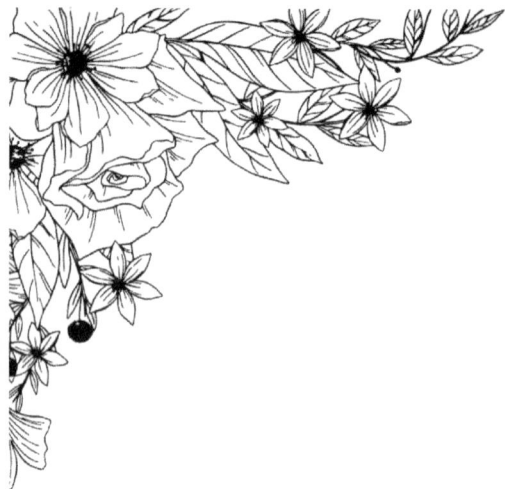

Yes, it is a great thing to invest financially.

But answer this, what have you gained if you forget to invest in your whole self?

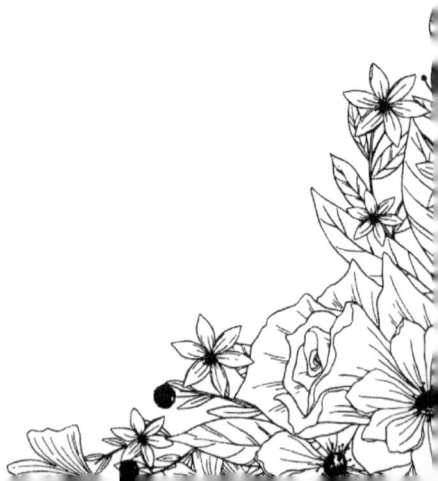

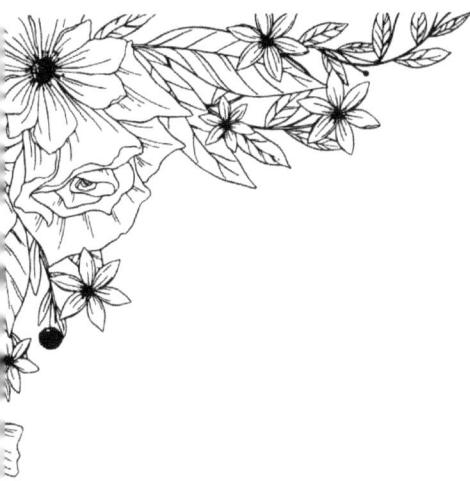

Stop waiting on someone to save you,

save yourself.

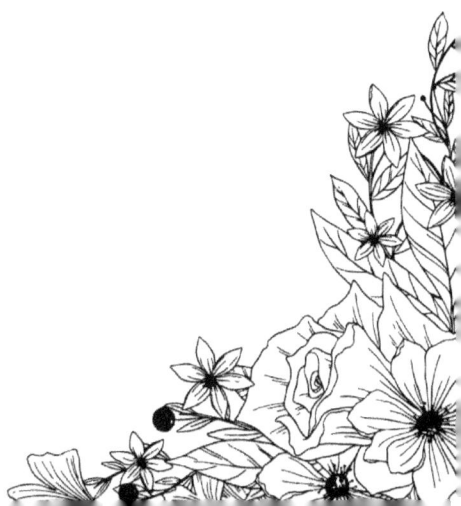

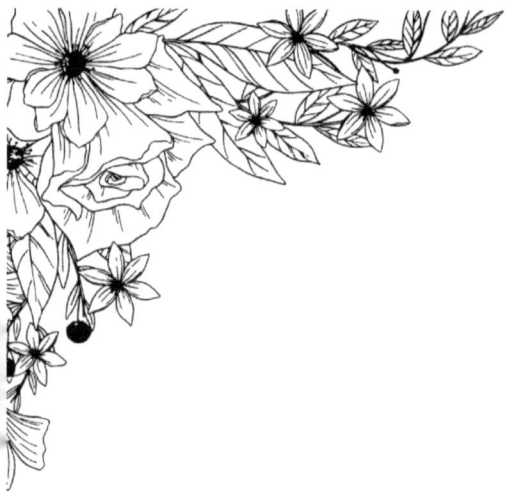

There comes a time when you realize you are worth everything someone made you feel like you were not!

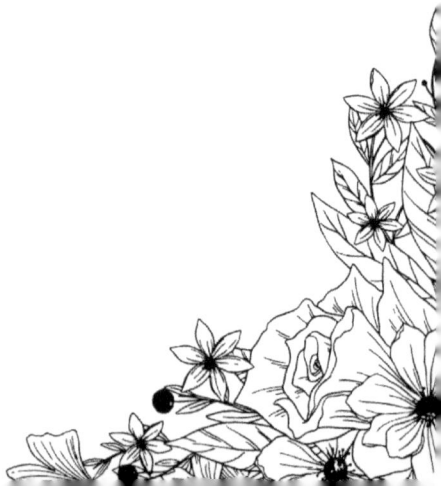

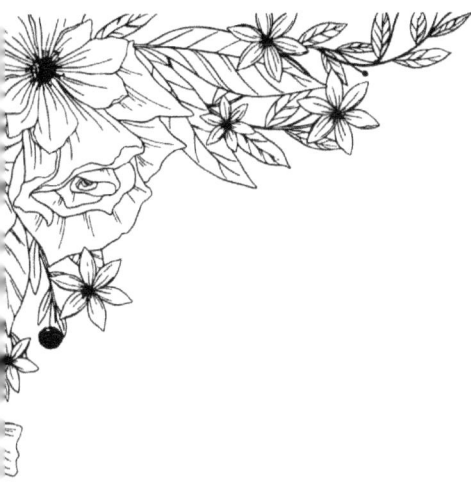

Being single may be hard but so is being in a relationship with someone who does not love you.

Choose your hard!

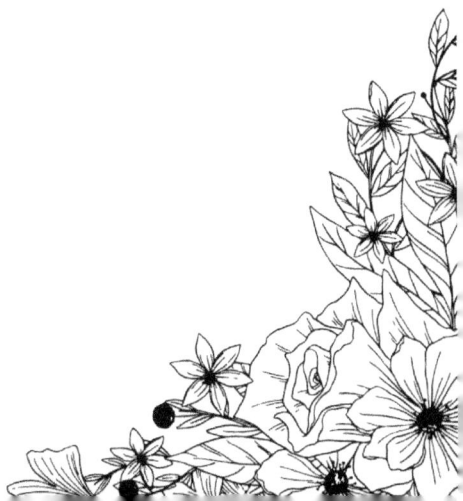

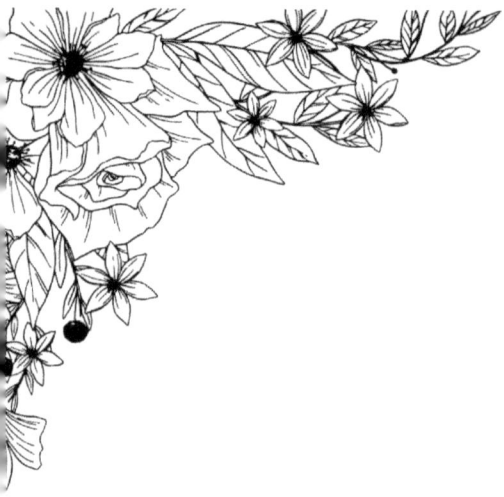

Do not fill your space with just anything/anyone
simply because you are lonely!

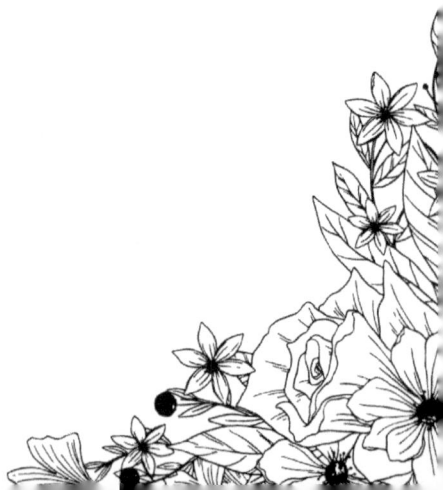

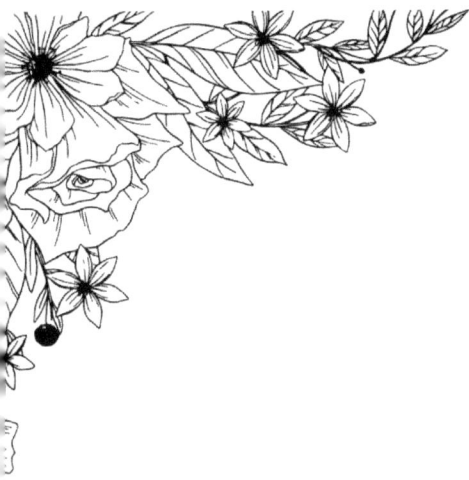

Stop caring about those who do not care about you!
Preserve that energy.

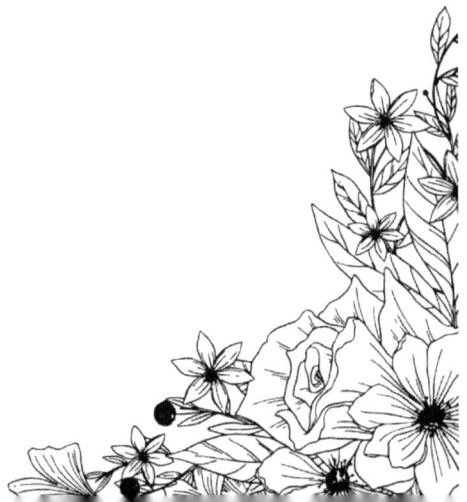

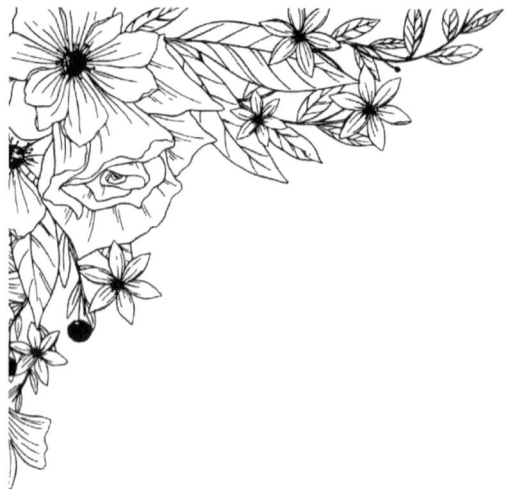

There is only one you, protect yourself.

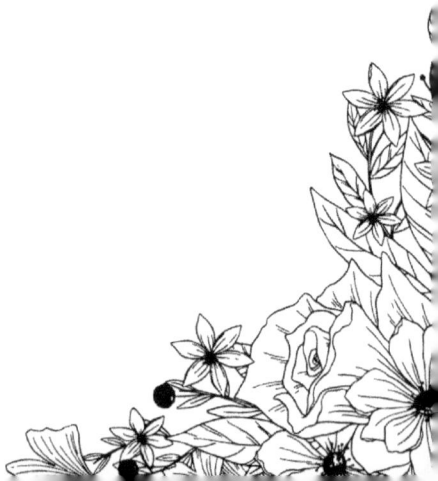

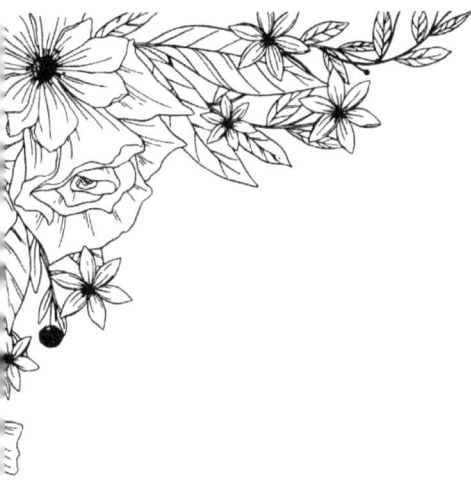

No one is allowed to tell you how to heal!

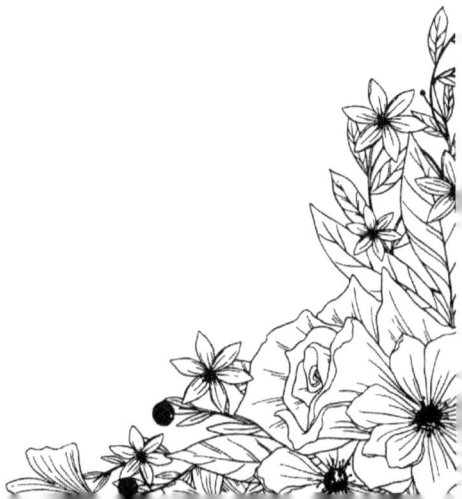

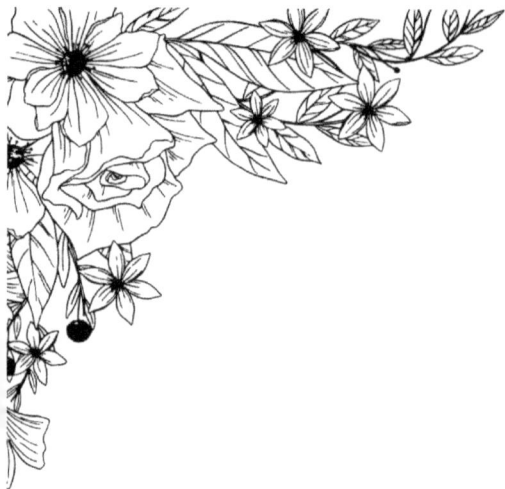

Your future will resemble your past, if you continue
to utilize the same blueprint.

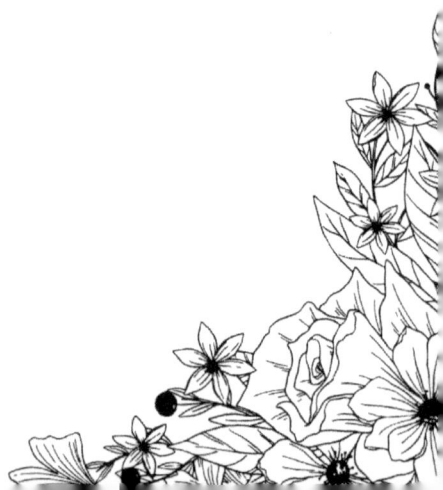

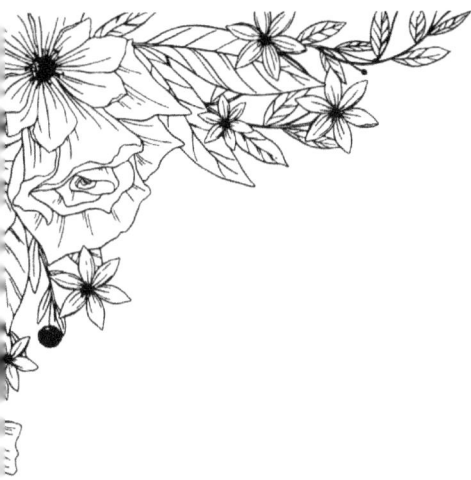

People will laugh at your standards when they have none of their own.

Do not lower them for anyone.

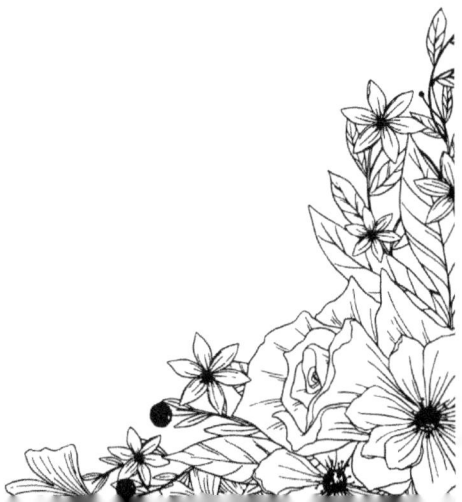

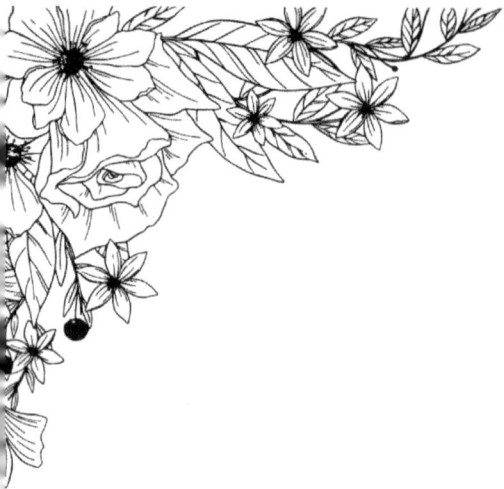

If you are everything to everyone else, what are you to yourself?

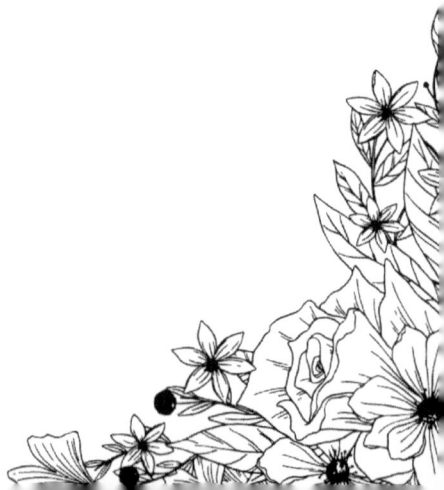

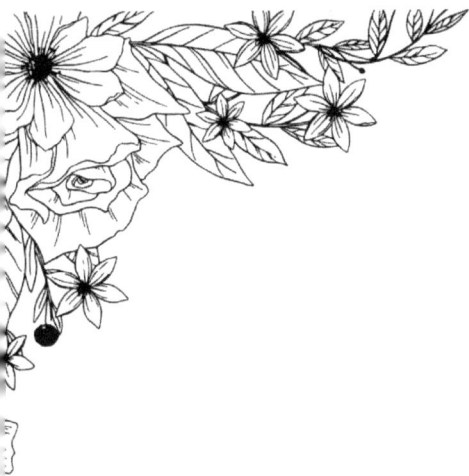

Stop minimizing your emotions and how you feel just so that others may feel "comfortable".

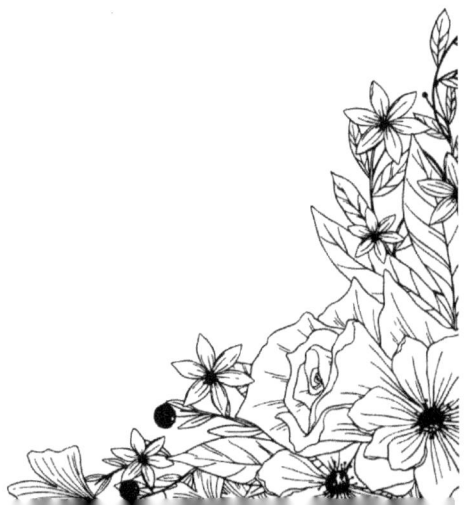

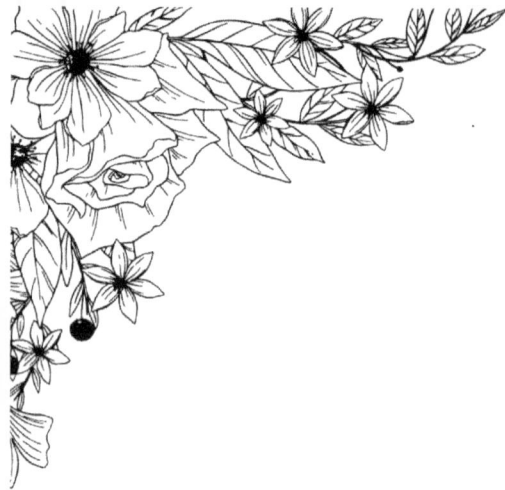

Focus on contentment not resentment.

Be happy with the life you have and let go of all the
negativity that no longer matters.

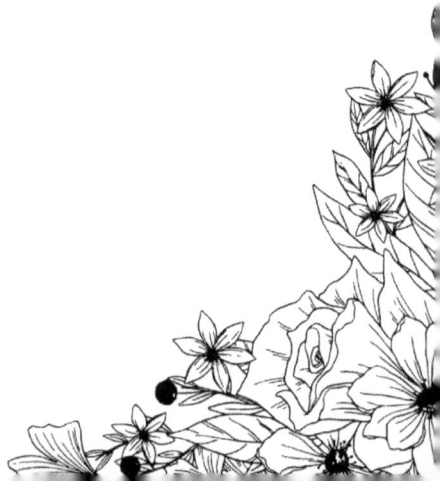

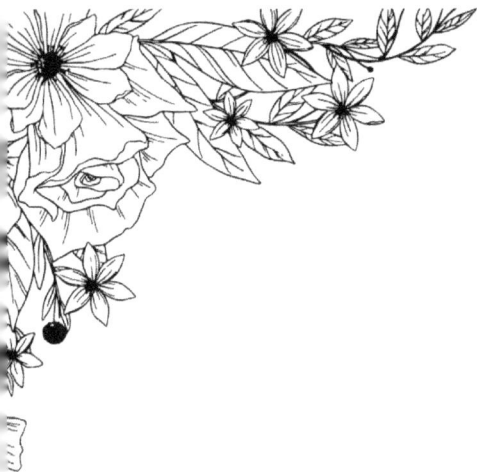

Not everyone deserves to be a character in your story.

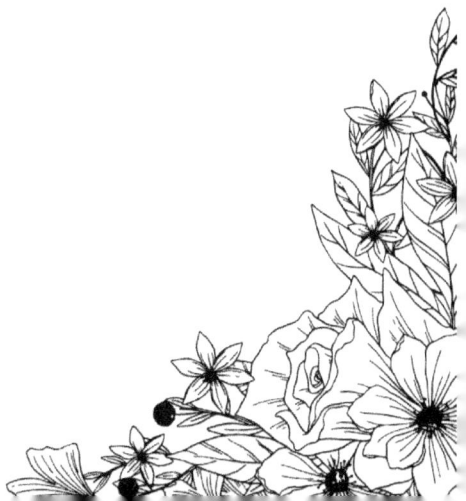

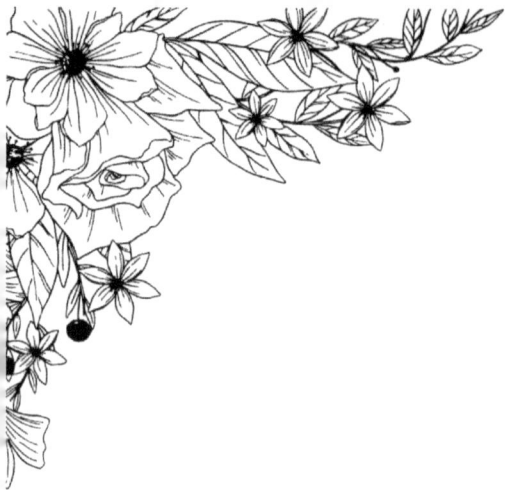

When a person cannot do something themselves, they will make you feel as though you cannot do it either. Do not believe them. You can do anything you want to do.

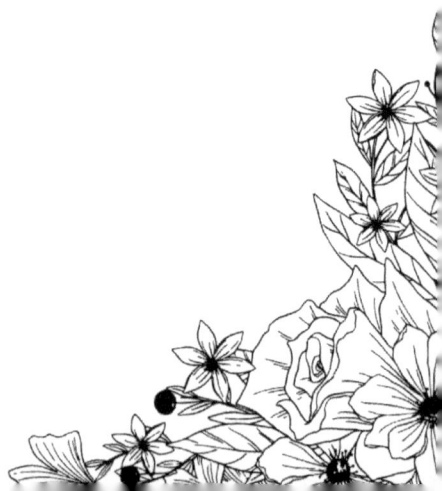

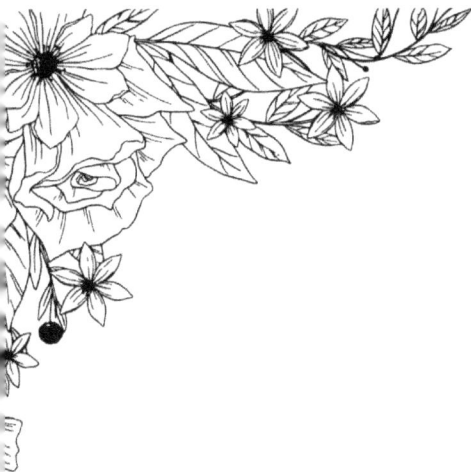

It is fine to look back on your past, but only when it is being used as an indicator of what not to do in your present and future.

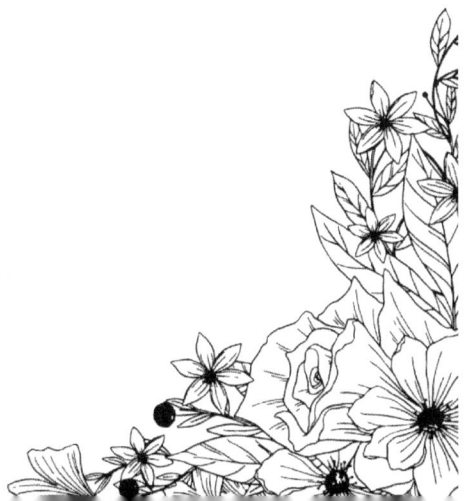

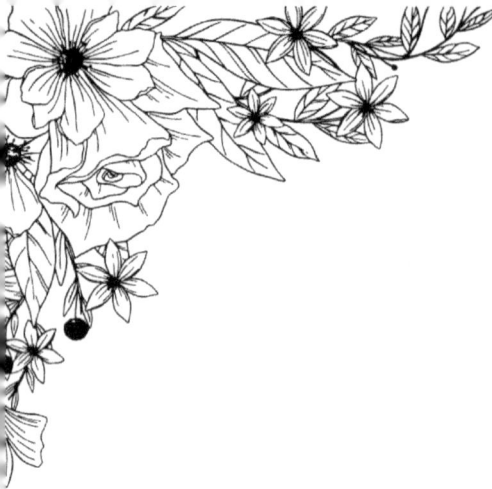

One should never compromise themselves so much that they lose who they are. Stay true to yourself, in relationships and life!

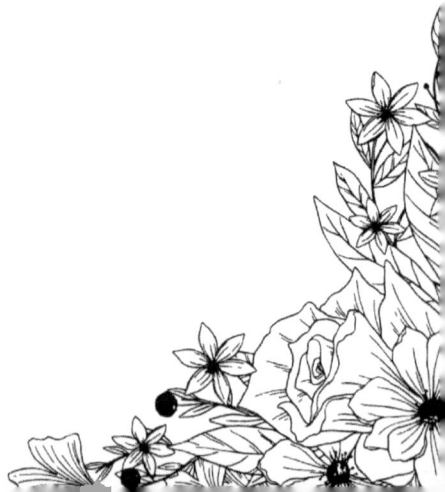

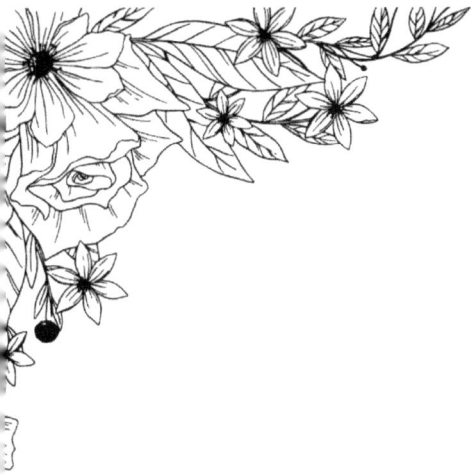

Do not gamble with your soul.

It is so hard to win back once you have lost it.

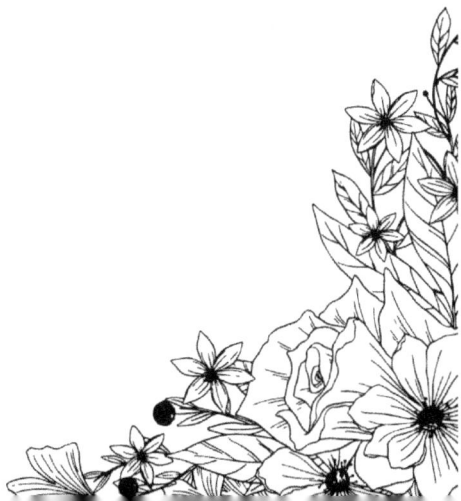

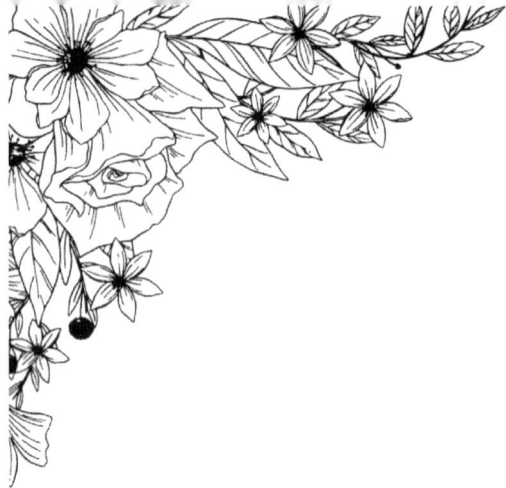

I became aware of what I deserved, fought for it,
and now no one can give me less.

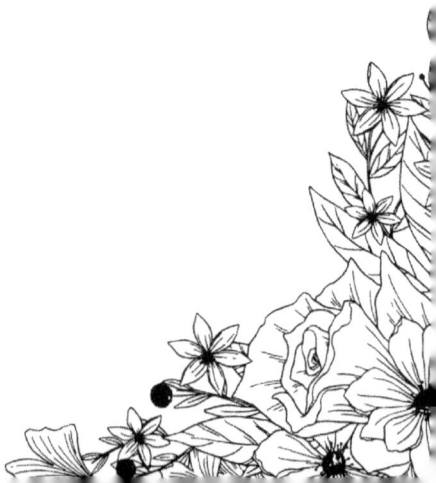

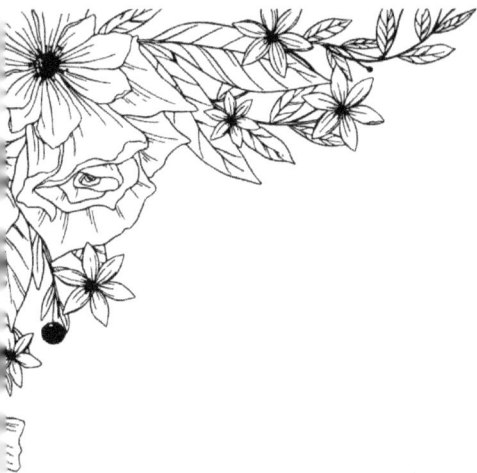

Do not give a person the power to break you when they were not the ONE who made you!

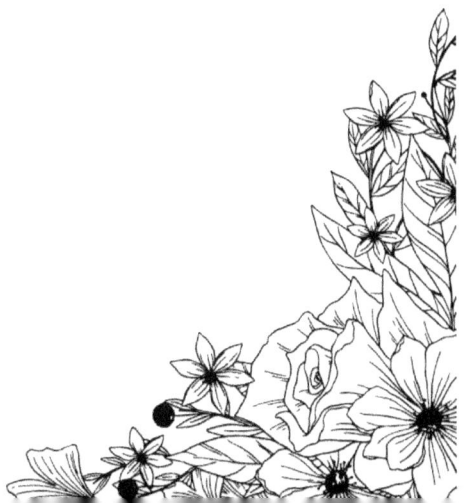

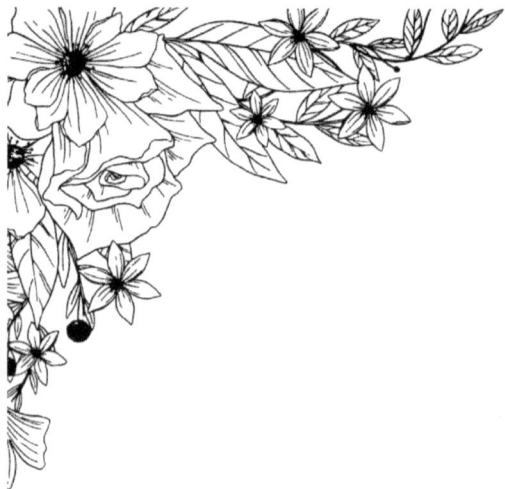

Stop getting in the way of your own happiness. You decide how you live, no one else.

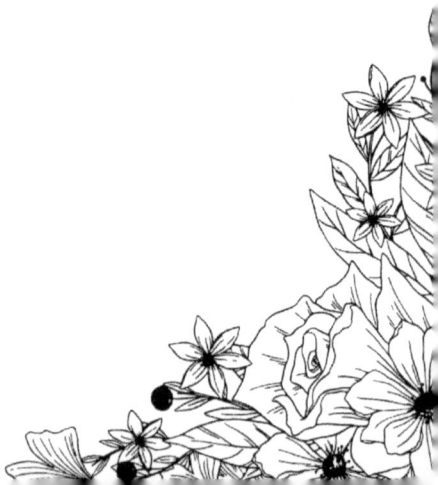

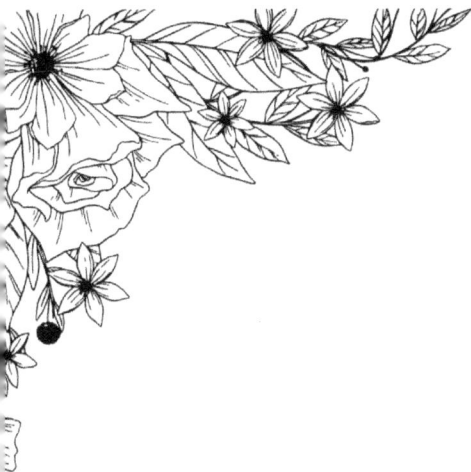

Time changes, and so do you.

Just like you cannot rush time, you also cannot rush progress.

Be patient with yourself, like you would want someone to be patient with you.

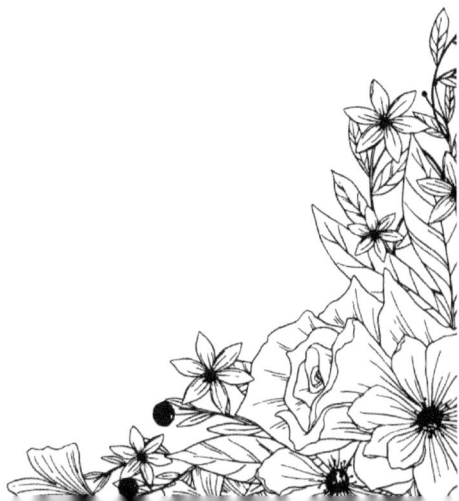

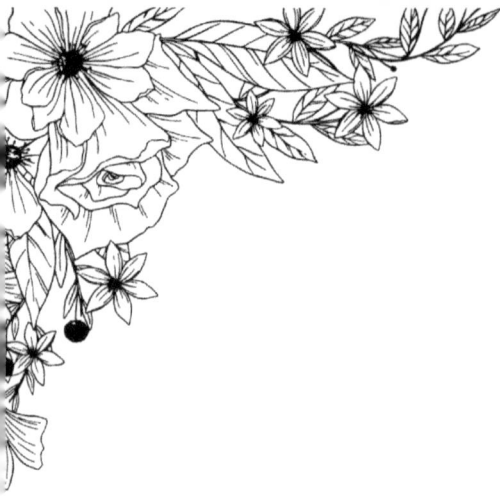

Most people will not value you the way you value them!

It is then time to move on.

Life is too short to always be wondering who is there for you!

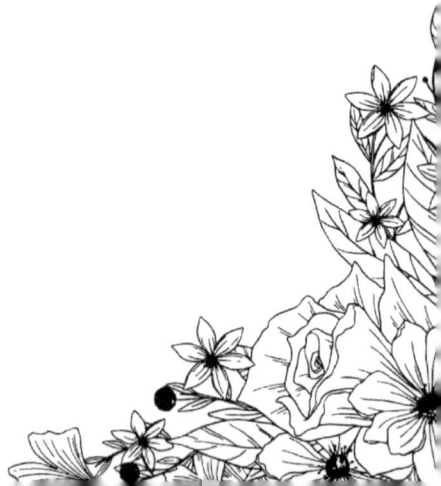

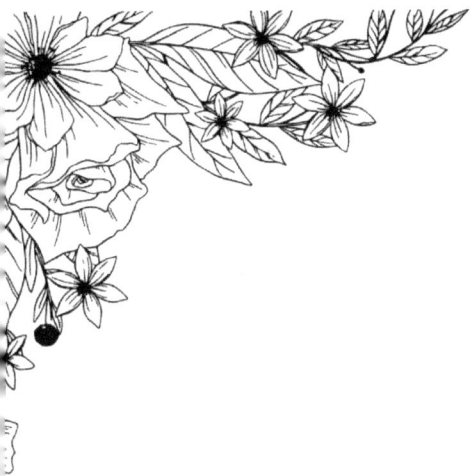

I see love in your eyes, for the first time in your whole life, and you are the one who put it there.

Self-love looks good on you!

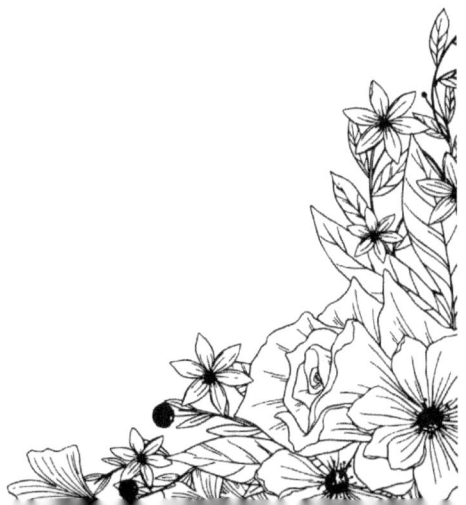

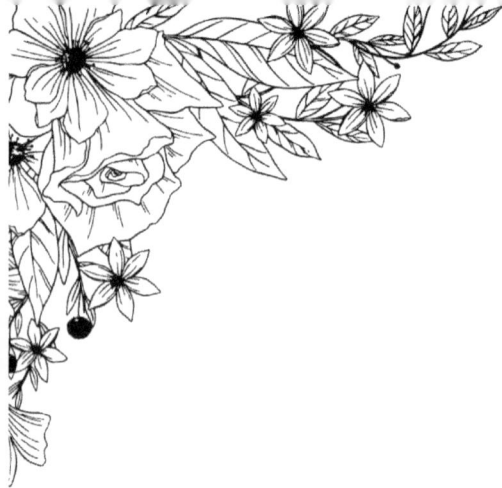

Do not allow someone who does not even belong in your present to mess up your future.

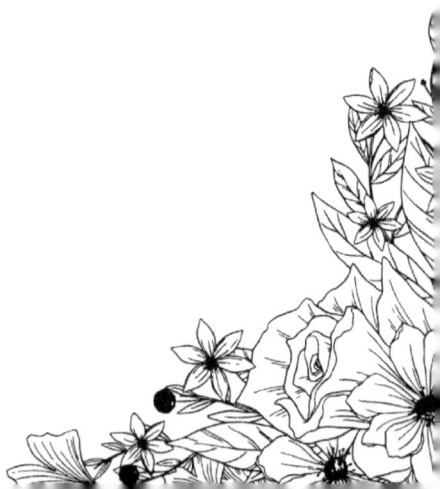

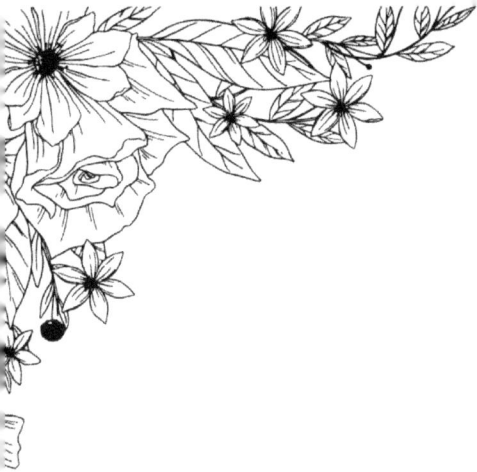

Stop making excuses for people who treat you badly.

There is no excuse!

You deserve the best, so quit accepting the worst.

I have said it before, and I will say it again. Life has taught me that if you give someone unlimited chances to hurt you, they will take every chance.

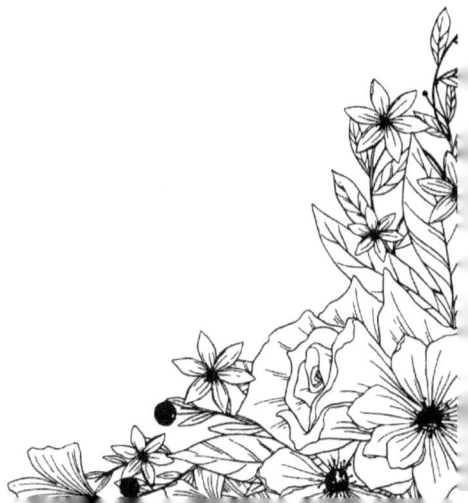

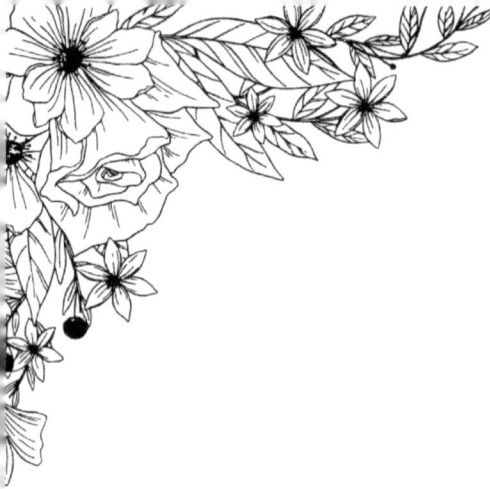

Love hard, but smart. Be good to each other, and most importantly be good to yourself!

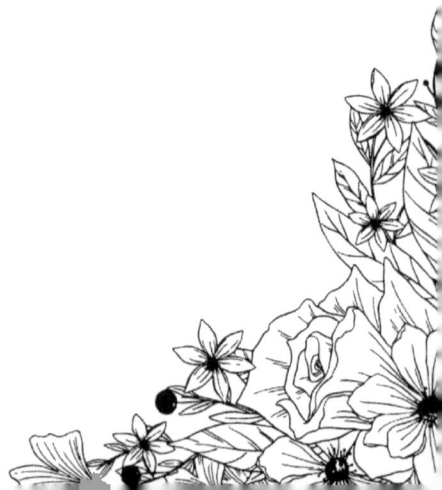

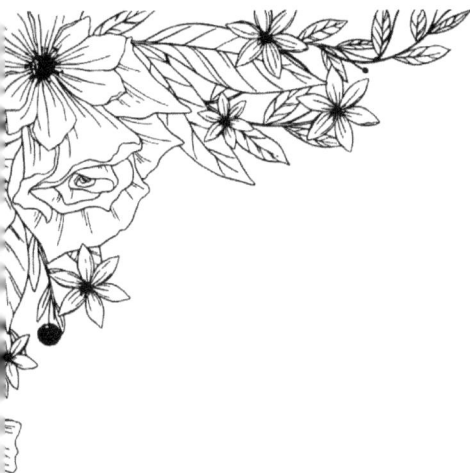

I hope you find what you are looking for because I did!

I absolutely love what I found, within myself.

Hopefully, you are that fortunate.

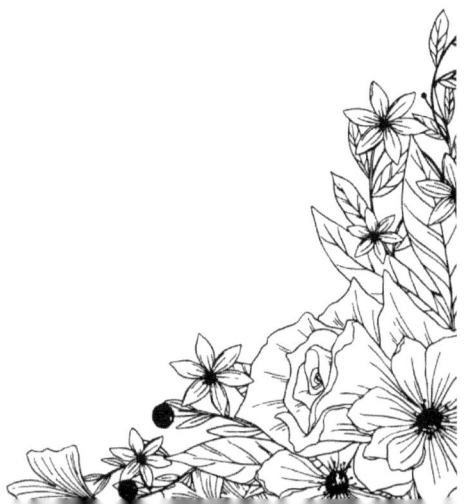

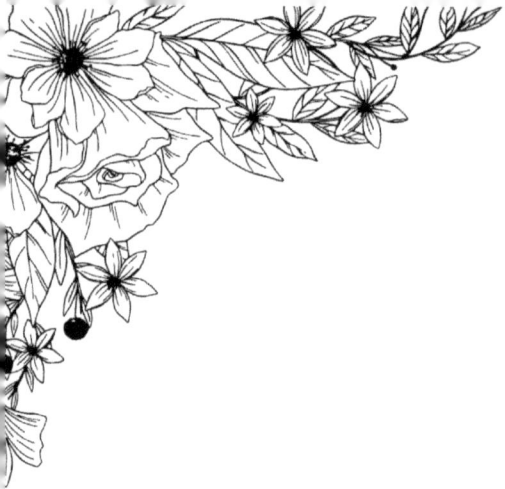

If a person does not respect themselves then they will not respect you.

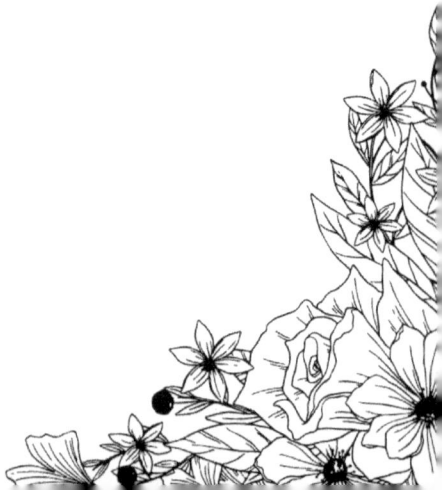

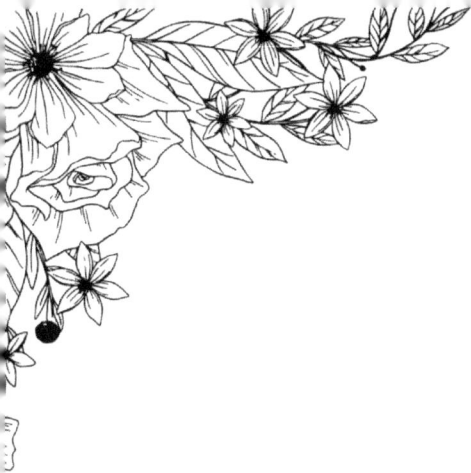

It is better to be with nobody and feel like somebody than to be with somebody and feel like nobody.

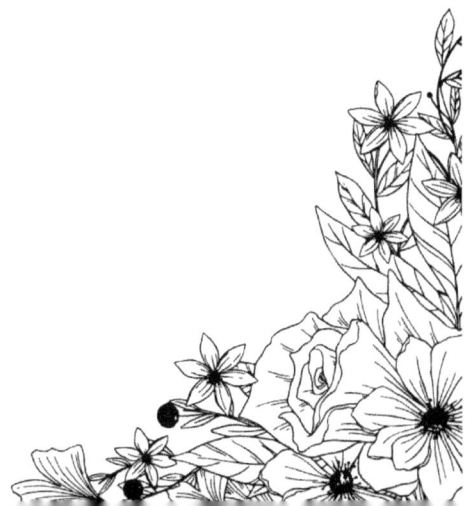

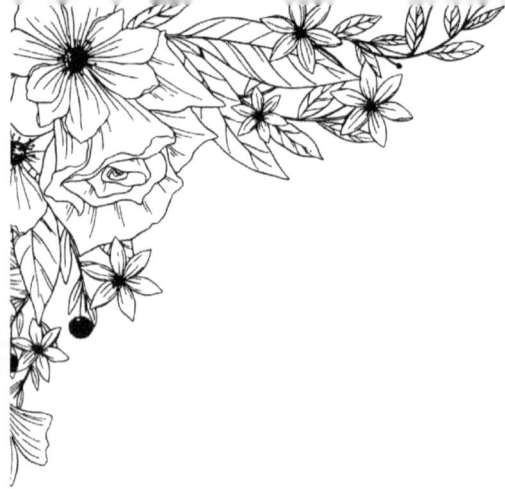

When the day is over and you have cared for everyone else, who is there to care for you?

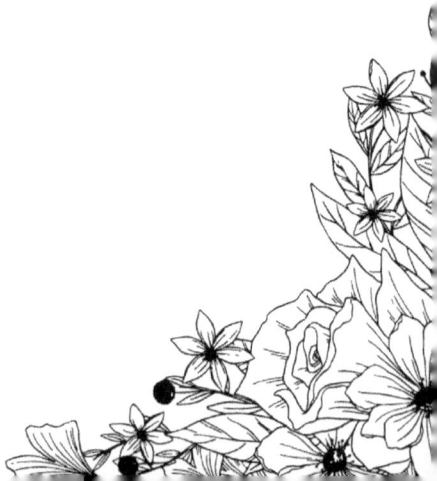

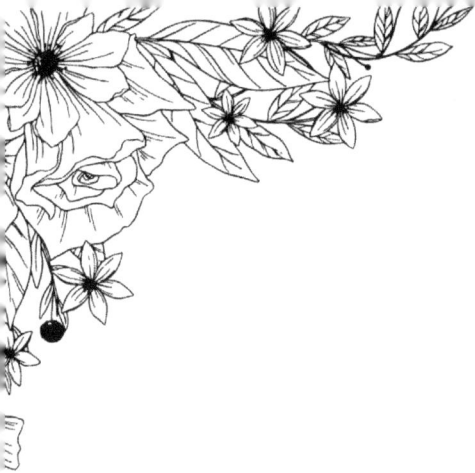

It is difficult to elevate when you are still in the same environment.

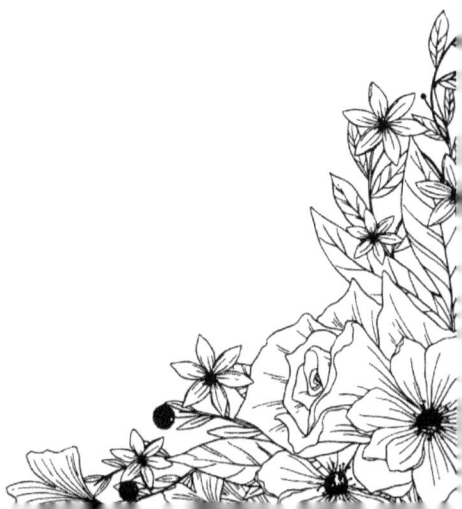

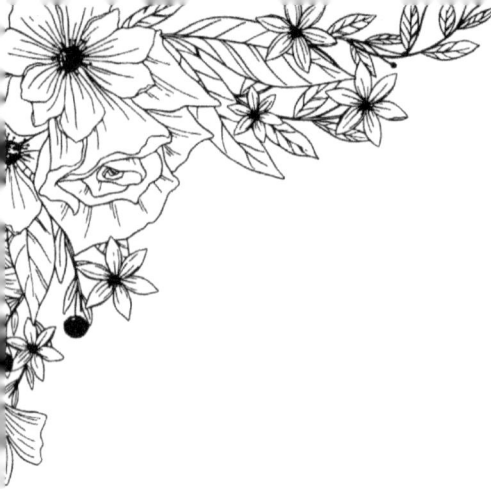

We are so used to asking others if they are okay, but how many times do we ask ourselves if we are okay?

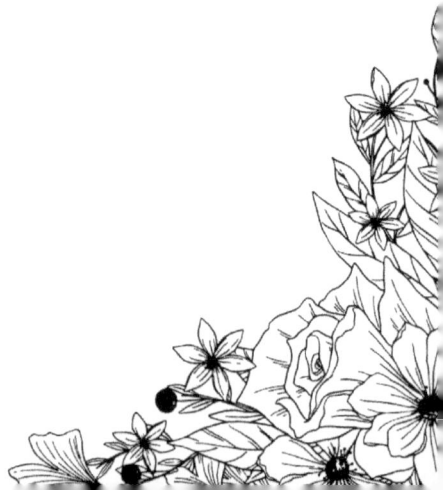

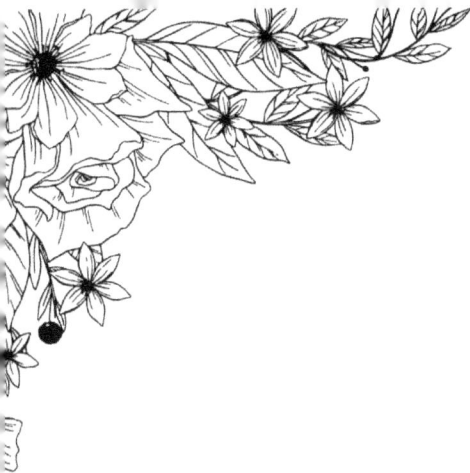

Stop allowing your past heartbreaks to interfere with your future happiness.

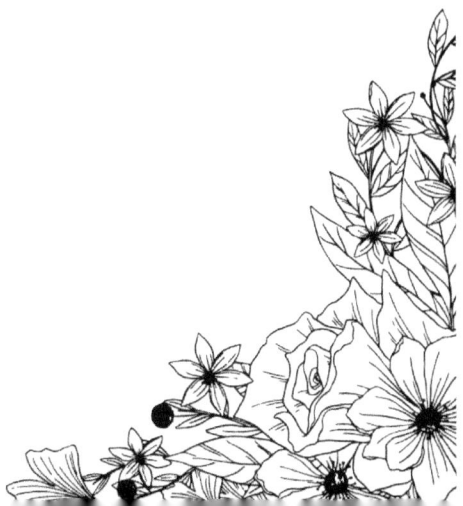

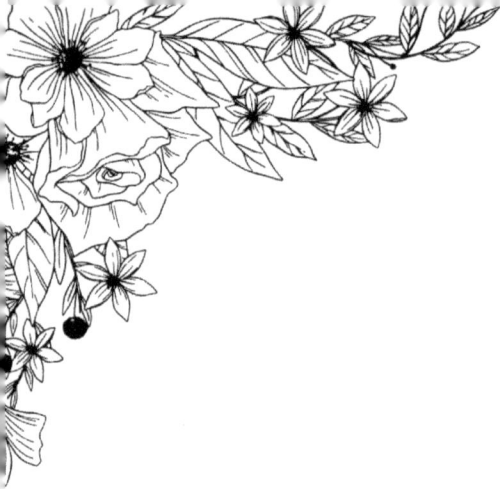

Be the comfort that you look for in others, to yourself.

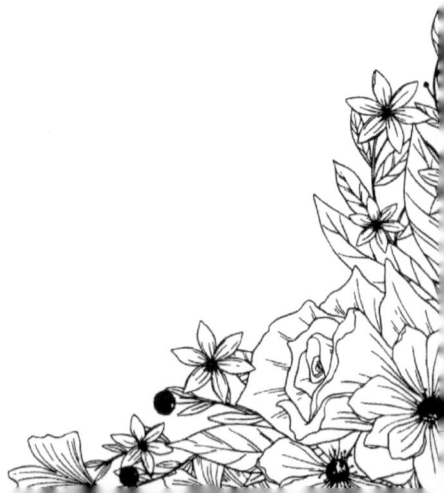

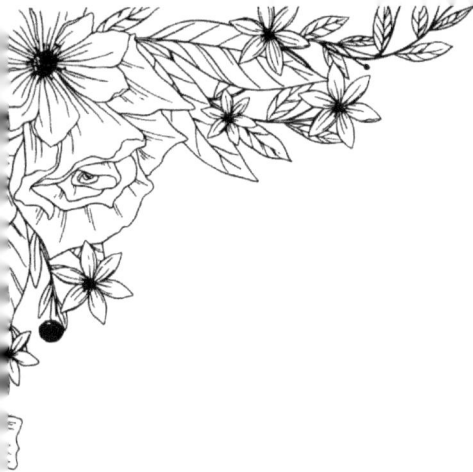

Mental vacations are just as important as physical vacations.

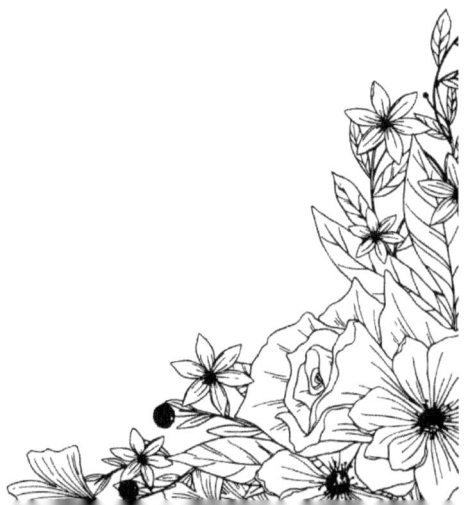

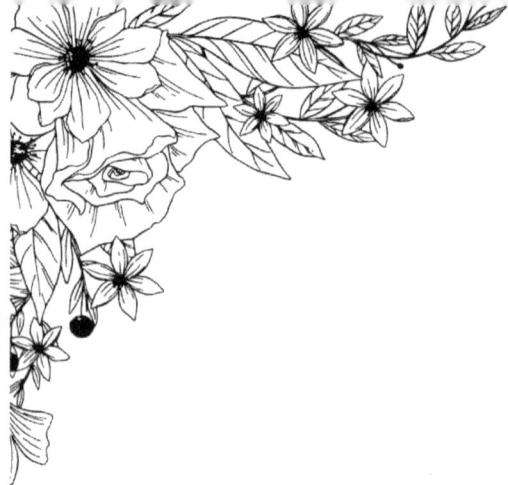

Look in the mirror and choose to love who you see.
You've been through a lot. You deserve to be loved,
and it starts with you!

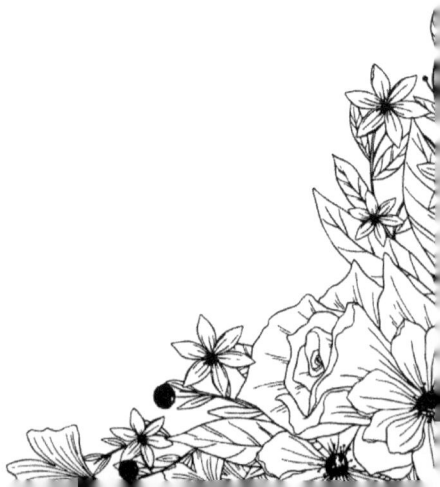

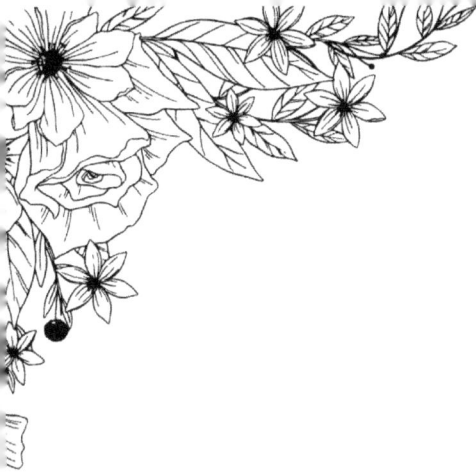

Let your confidence shine. Do not be ashamed that you know your worth!

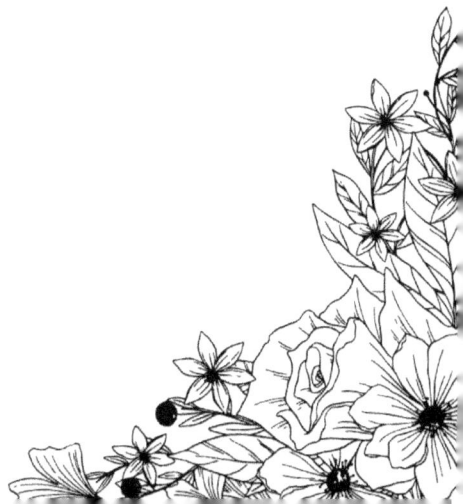

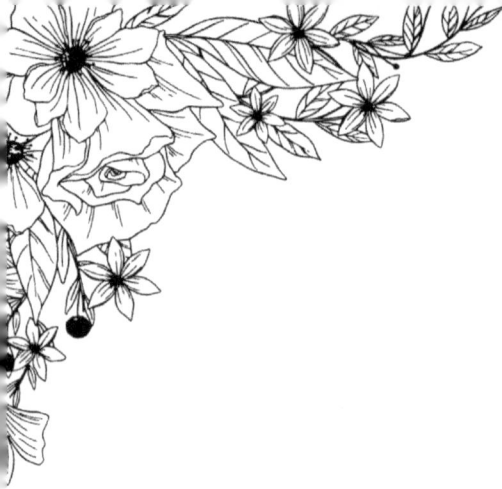

Be Free!

A lot of the fear we internalize is make believe.

I encourage you to do one thing that you are fearful of. You, more than you know, deserve to be free!

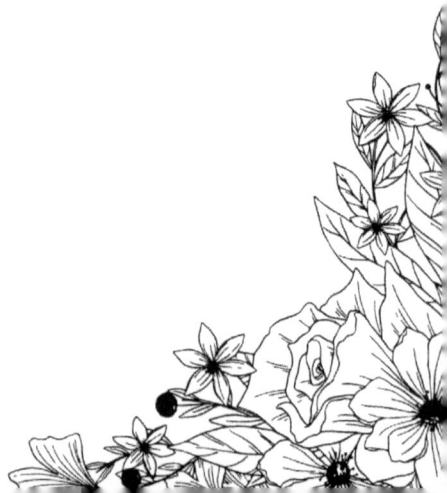

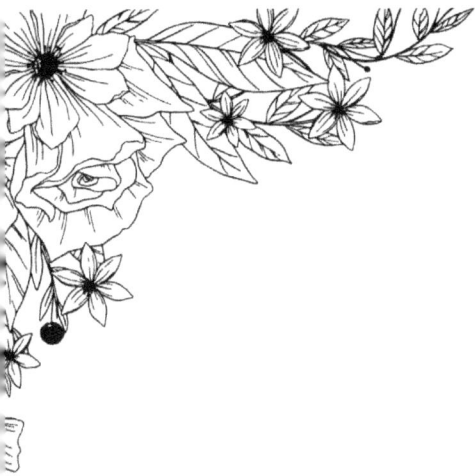

Loving someone who does not appreciate you is
like watering a fake plant.... USELESS.

Give your love to God, and He will return it with
such beauty and sincerity!

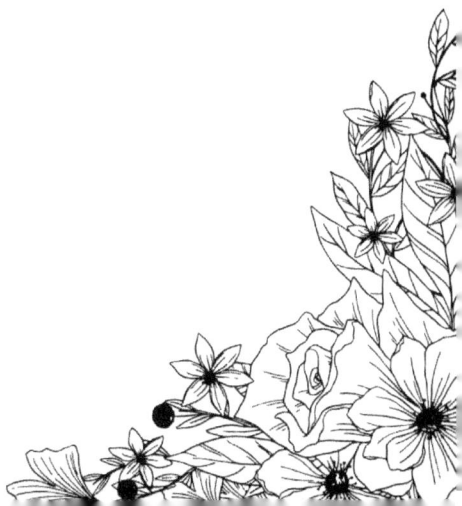

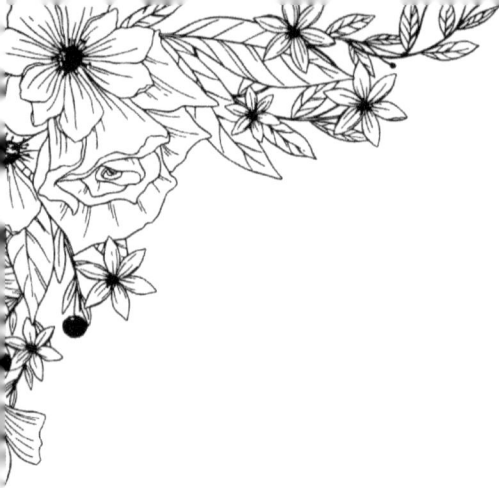

Often, we choose to run from our past and pretend like it does not exist.

However, if we are being honest, our past shapes the present us.

There are experiences that we expected to happen, but they did not.

Those are considered losses, and losses deserve to be mourned.

I encourage you to mourn, heal, move on, and love yourself!

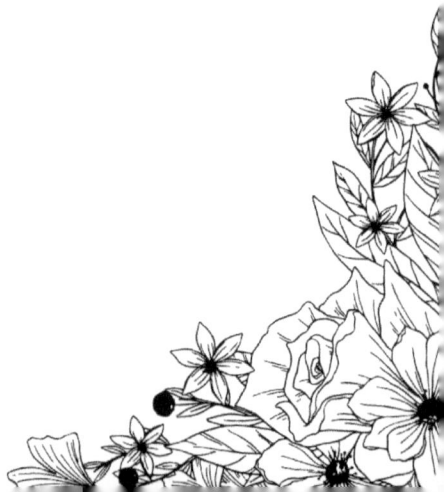

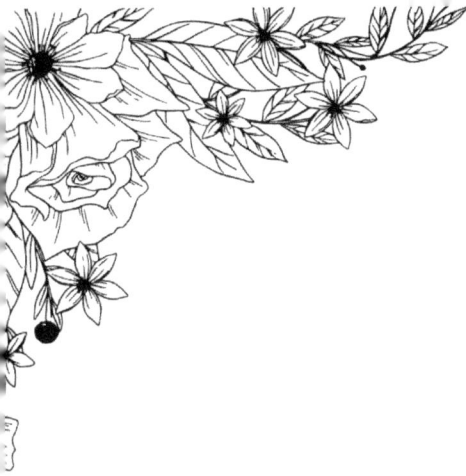

At my big old age, there is an inner child in me, and she loves adventure. Rollercoasters are my favorite thing, but only the ones found in amusement parks.

I genuinely have no desire to get on the emotional ones anymore.

The older I get, the more I realize that emotional rollercoasters no longer feel like adventure to me, like they did in my teenage years and my twenties.

Those rollercoasters feel like deliriously insane torture.

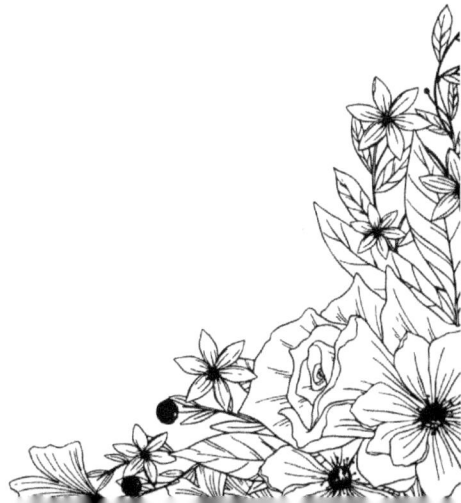

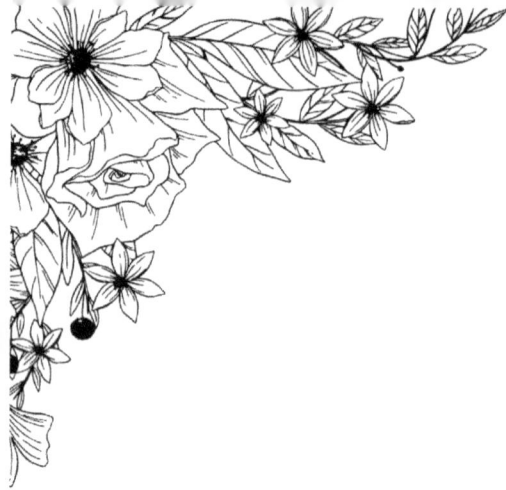

Do not let a person tell you more than once that they do not want you. Listen to them, the FIRST time.

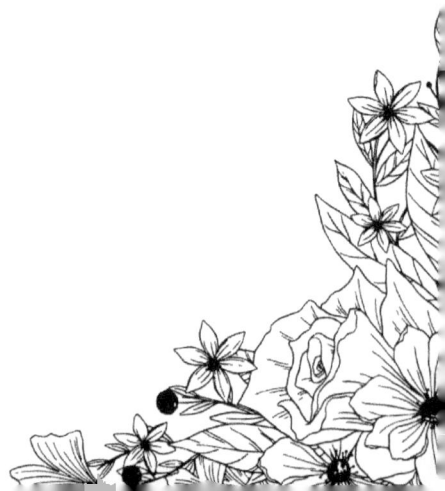

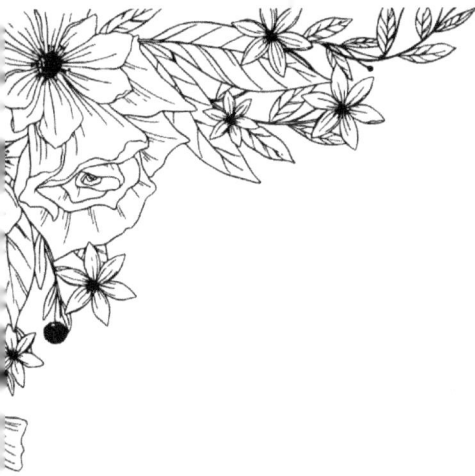

We all claim that we want freedom until we have it.

Then we self-sabotage and bond ourselves to people, places, and things.

Stop bonding yourself and be free.

You deserve freedom more than you know.

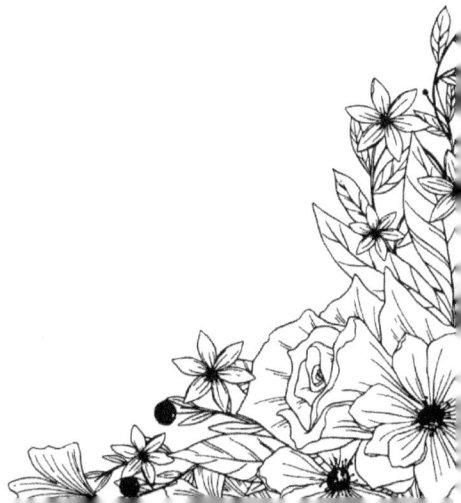

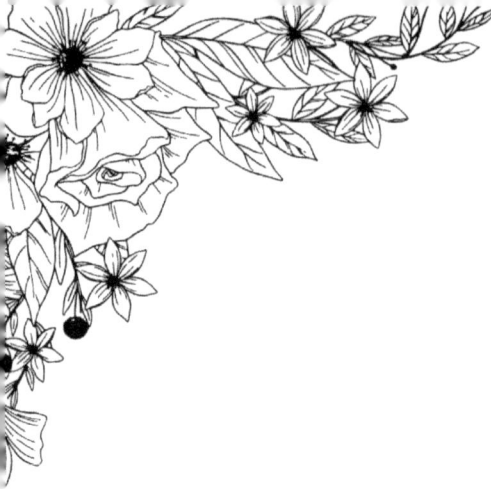

Self-love is taking care of my whole self. Self-love is not allowing others to make me feel like I'm not worthy. Self-love is taking care of my mental. Self-love is not allowing people to define me. Self-love is making sure I am safe! Self-love is giving myself permission to care for myself.

To me self-love is caring for myself in totality and not expecting or waiting around for others to do it!

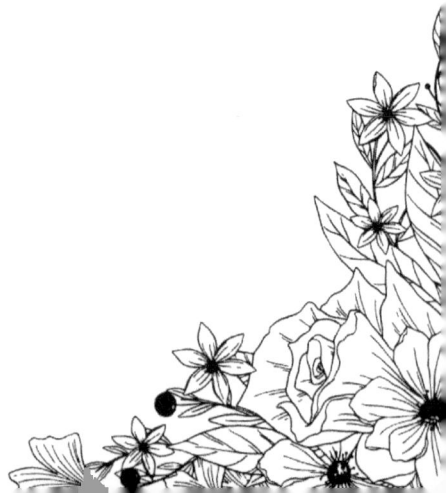

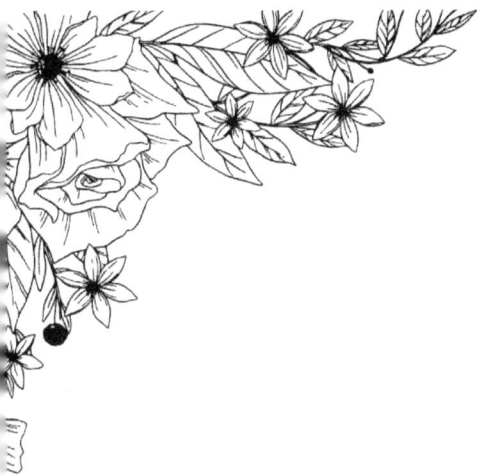

In a field of dreams, I found you.

You are love.

You are magnificent.

You are beautiful.

You are kind.

You are thoughtful.

You are impactful.

You matter.

You are ME!

In a field of dreams... I found myself!

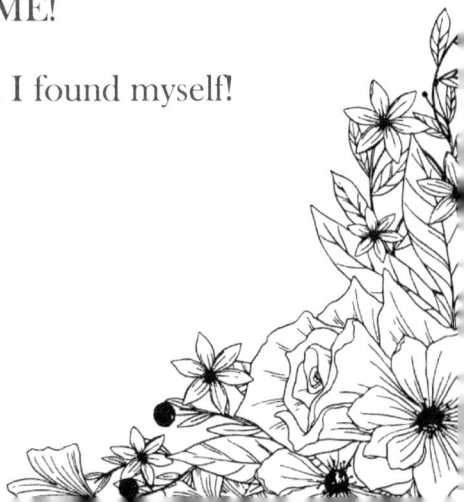

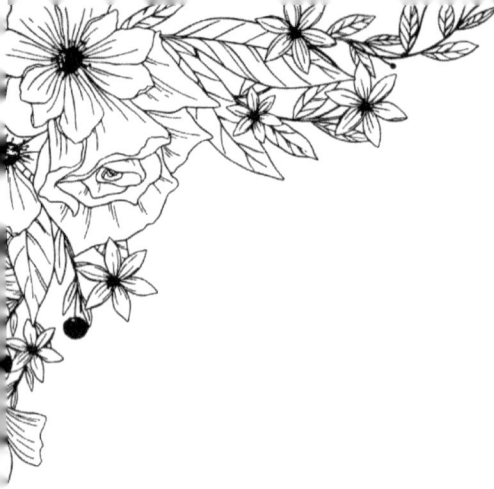

At the end of the day, I am just out here turning my losses into lessons and my brokenness into blessings.

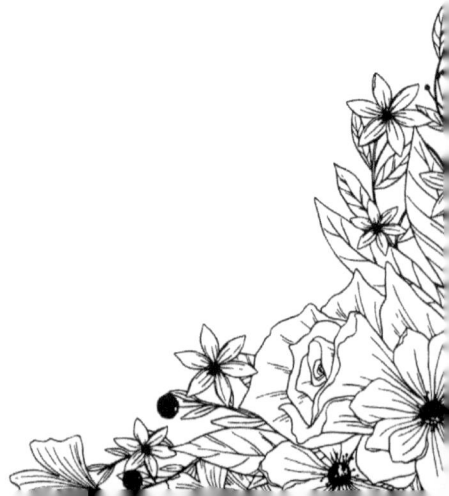

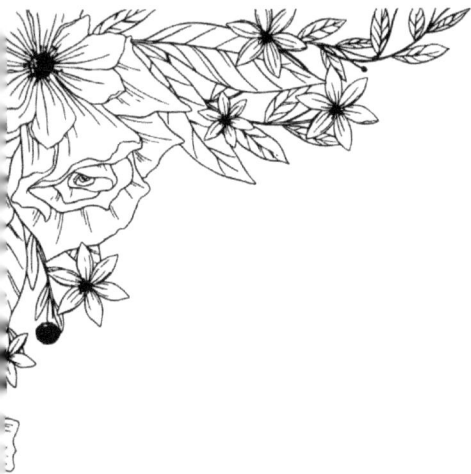

To quote one of my favorite songs, "You have got to trust the signs. Everything will turn out fine. So, why aren't you smiling?"

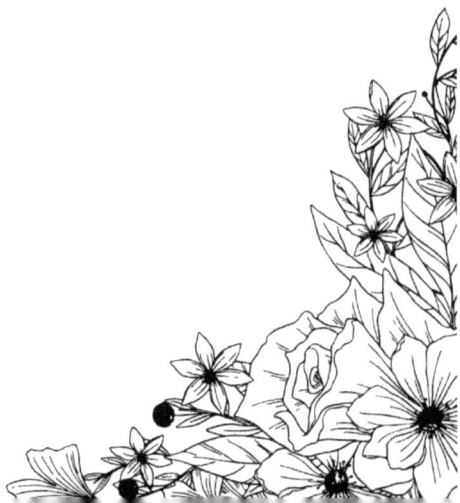

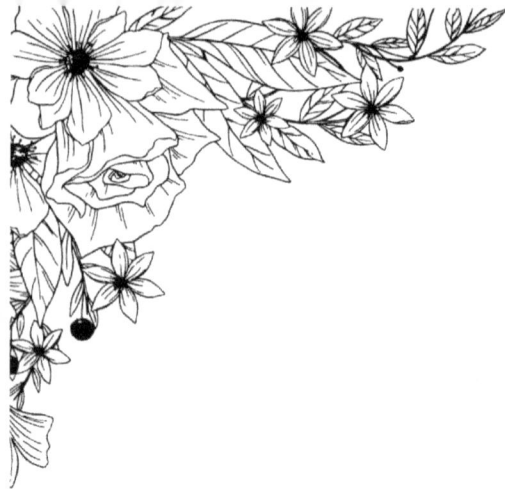

When we stop learning, we stop living. Everything has a lesson. EVERYTHING. While we may be unable to see the lesson at the time, it is there. When you finally see the lesson, it will all make sense. As I age, I am learning that I have gone through certain things to help others navigate their lives better. In the grand scheme of things, there are no real losses, when you are loving, just lessons. Keep living. Keep loving. Keep learning. One day it will all make sense.

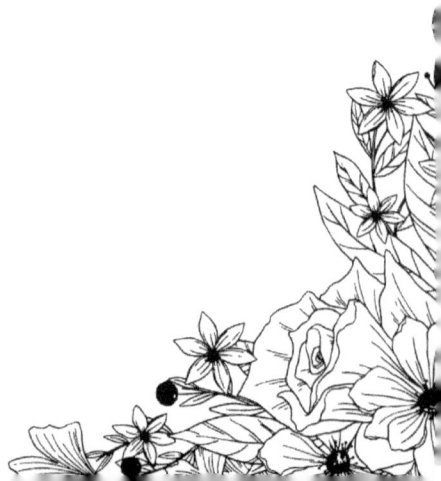

## Restart Yourself

When was the last time you restarted yourself? I mean physically closed down, did some inner work, and came back refreshed?

To be honest it has been a while for me, but I thought... "if my phone needs to be restarted, and it does not do half of the work I do, then maybe I need to restart myself too!"

• •

If our technology glitches, then what makes us think that we do not glitch?

What makes us think that we do not need moments to just not always be ON?

• •

It is important that we take time away - take time off! Because if we ignore our warnings to restart, eventually we will shut down, and WE DO NOT NEED THAT!

• •

So, this is the sign you were looking for. Take that break, go on that vacation, put your phone on DND, just do what you need to do to restart!

Write a letter to your ex/exes!

• •

Hear me out! HEAR. ME. OUT!

YOU DO NOT HAVE TO SEND IT!

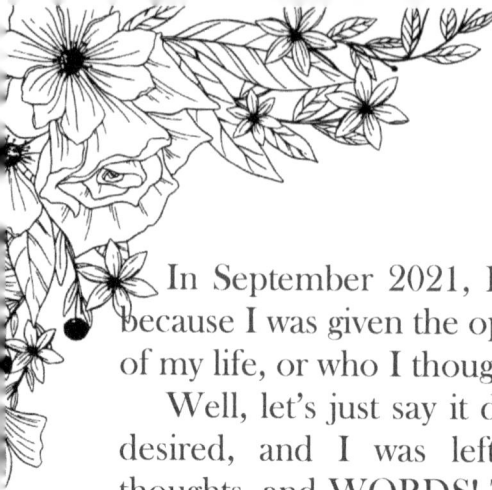

In September 2021, I reached a real low point because I was given the opportunity to meet the love of my life, or who I thought was the love of my life.

Well, let's just say it did not end in a way that I desired, and I was left with so many feelings, thoughts, and WORDS! Things I could not tell this person because they did not want to hear me, and they DID NOT care about me or my words. Well, what was I supposed to do with these emotions, these words?! Where could I put them?

• •

As I sat crying in my hands, something hit me to write a letter to my ex, not only this ex, but ALL of them! Once I put that pen to paper, my soul became lighter and lighter. I said what I wanted to say without being interrupted or misunderstood, and that gave me more closure than I have EVER received from talking to an ex.

• •

This may seem like a lot to do, but if you have a specific ex or exes that are still tugging at your heart and soul, but you have no contact with them, I implore you to write them a letter to get all your words out. You deserve this closure and freedom!

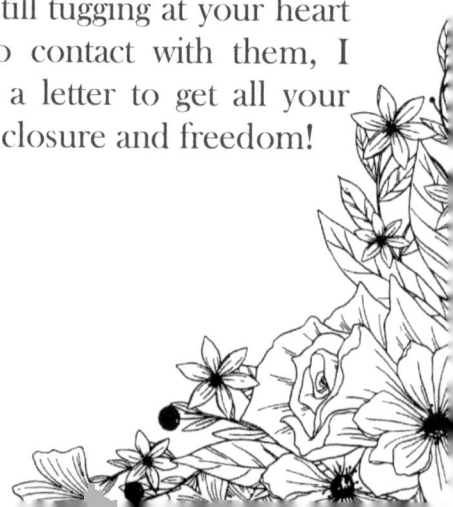

# MENTAL HEALTH IS BEAUTIFUL!

Sometimes I cannot hear myself think, and sometimes ALL I can hear is myself think. One day I am on Mount Everest, and the next day I am in the Challenger Deep! I can smile in immense pain, and I can cry in delirious happiness. I can be completely calm or completely frantic.

My #MentalHealth struggles are Attention Deficit/Hyperactivity Disorder, depression, and anxiety. While I have learned to manage it and love it, I still struggle at times. I have had ADHD since elementary school (it is not as prevalent as it was in my adolescence), and I was diagnosed with Major Depressive Disorder when I was 18 years old!

[[OH MY WORD! Did an African American woman just admit she has depression? Alert the ancestors, she is not allowed to talk about this!]]

When I received the MDD diagnosis, it came with a friend, Polycystic Ovarian Syndrome or PCOS. This disorder is what caused me to have Depression and Anxiety. It is the reason I cannot sleep some nights. It is the reason I can go a million miles a minute until I crash. It is the reason why sometimes I cannot breathe until I am able to break down and cry! It is... my superpower.

As I grew older, I realized that Mental Health is real. I realized that it did not make a person "CRAZY"; it made them unique. What people do not understand is Depression, Bipolar Disorder, Schizophrenia Disorder,

Disorder, Personality Disorders, etc looks different with each person who has been diagnoses with any of the aforementioned diagnoses. Even when given a general label, there is still uniqueness in that person.

I speak about Mental Health because you cannot live, love, or listen if you do not know about Mental Health! I have always wanted to help others. That is my lifelong goal. Long story short, I wanted to be a Lawyer, but I ended up becoming a Social Worker. I landed right in the middle of the Mental Health field, and I know it was only God who placed me there. As I studied and learned about Mental Health and Mental Illnesses, it baffled me to find out that African American people suffered too. In our culture, we are told to pray and seek God, and while I believe He is the only way to make it through, I knew I needed something in addition to His perfection.

I needed therapy.

In the summer of 2018, I began therapy. I began therapy because I knew that while I prayed and sought God, He was leading me to therapy. I needed to scream. I needed to yell. I needed to feel safe. I found safety and acceptance in therapy.

It is okay to go to therapy. I REPEAT: IT IS OKAY TO GO TO THERAPY. It does not make you crazy. It does not make you insane. It makes you smart and aware.

Therapy was a life saver.

Due to my allotted number of sessions finishing, and my desire to get therapy from someone who looks like me, I found a new therapist in 2020. I have to say that before I went to therapy, I had already started working on my life, internally. I was doing self-care, taking myself on dates, and reading affirmations and positive quotes, daily! I began meditating and doing breathing exercises.

The truthful reason why I went to therapy, I was not properly dealing with the past rapes that have happened in my life. Those occurrences coupled with depression are a recipe for disaster. When I say it is SO vital to check in mentally, it is! If I had continued living in a state of denial, I probably would not be here.

I say all that to say, if you have been diagnosed with a mental illness.. YOU ARE NOT INSANE. YOU ARE NOT CRAZY. YOU ARE AN AMAZING INDIVIDUAL who needs a little extra help in life. That is nothing to be ashamed of. Speak up! Tell others, you have more support than you believe. I would not be where I am without my support system! Never forget, your #MentalHealthIs BEAUTIFUL!

Healing is not something you do just to check it off of your "to do" list. Healing is a journey that requires you to feel emotions that may break your heart again. It is sitting in those emotions and then growing from them, until they no longer cause you pain! We, as humans, live in a society where we want EVERYTHING fast, so we think we can pop our healing into a microwave -microwave for four minutes and then we are healed! Sorry, it does not work like that! Healing takes patience, acknowledgment, grace, forgiveness (for you and them), and MORE PATIENCE! Be patient with yourself. It is okay to mourn the loss of the relationship. It is okay to mourn the loss of yourself. It is okay to mourn the loss of your former partner! While we are mourning, do not forget to continue healing! To be healed is a beautiful thing, and so is the journey - do not rush it, you may miss something important!

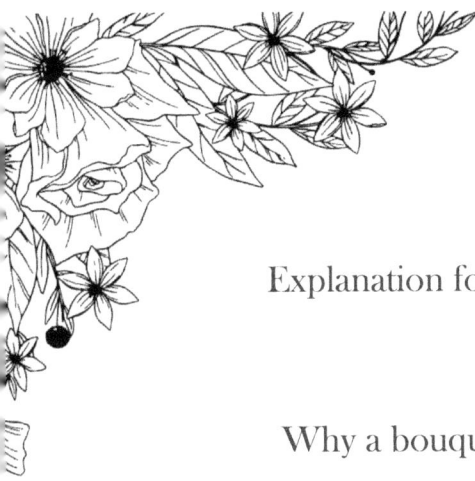

Explanation for my cover art:

Why a bouquet of flowers?

So, I was in a relationship with someone for some years (the relationship right before my self-love journey), and I would always bring up that I love flowers, and he would always make an excuse about why he wasn't getting them. His favorite excuse was... "they are too expensive."

So, me being the researcher I am, said "no, you can get them for $10 at Walmart!"

He then rebutted with, "there are $5 roses at Kroger."

I responded with, "See! I would love those too."

• •

Years later, I remember what he said like it was yesterday.

• •

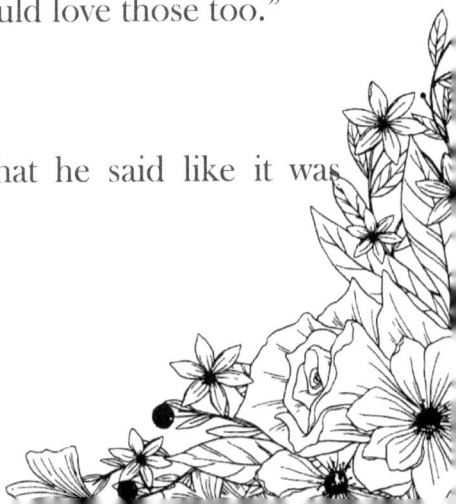

237

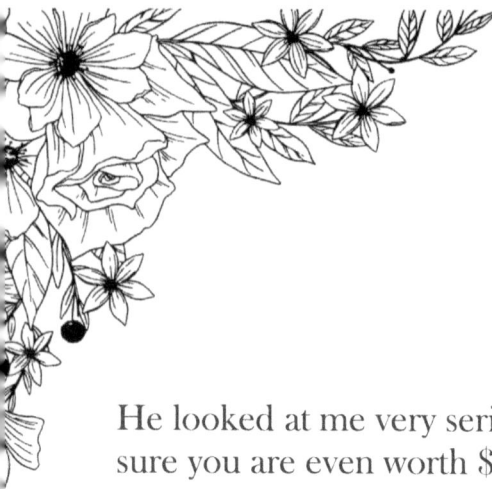

He looked at me very seriously, and said, "I'm not sure you are even worth $5 flowers.

Needless to say, it ended a few months after that. I was broken + believed I was worthless, so I didn't know to leave sooner. Psychological abuse is REAL, especially when you've been with someone for years!

• •

When the relationship ended, that same day, the first thing I went out and bought were flowers.

• •

Now I buy myself flowers often!

It's a beautiful reminder that I'm worth all the things I deprived myself of while being in toxic relationships!

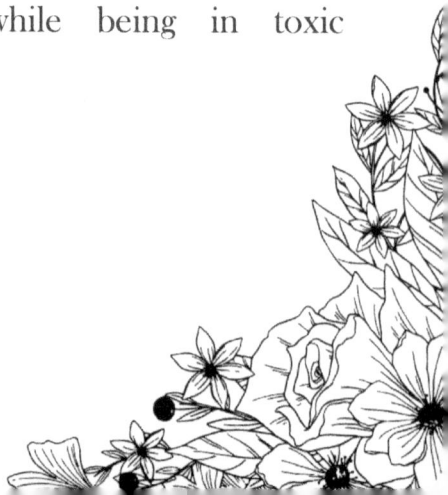

• •

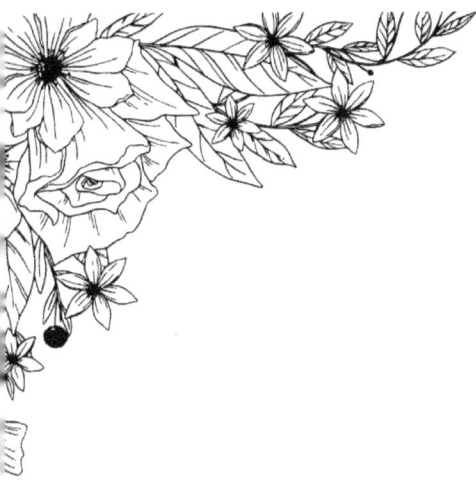

Do Not Allow Someone To Half Love You!!

You are kind.

You are beautiful.

You are worthy.

YOU ARE ENOUGH!

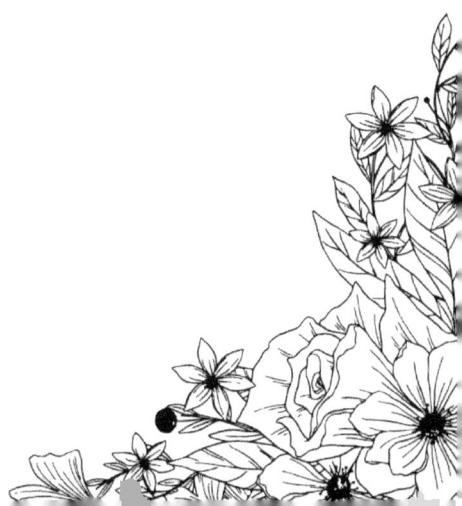

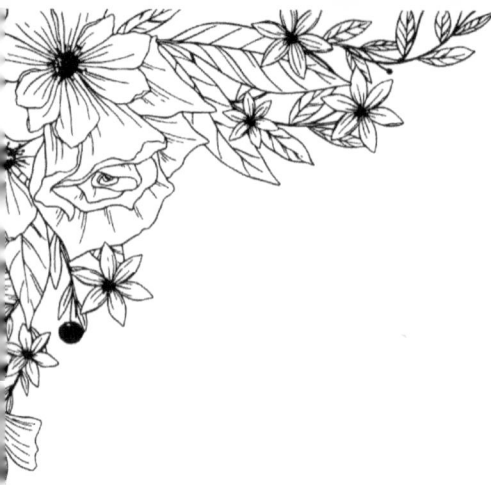

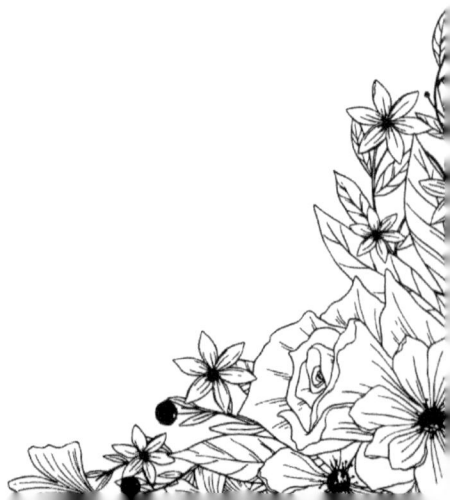

www.ingramcontent.com/pod-product-compliance
Lightning Source LLC
Chambersburg PA
CBHW052110030426

42335CB00025B/2926